Rolling With It:

A Guide to Living and

Thriving with a Disability

Lucy May Neat-Ward

Disclaimers

Please note that all information regarding schemes/ laws such as the Equality Act 2010, DSA, PIP, Access to Work, Motability, NHS Wheelchair Services and other schemes was correct at time of publication [31 October 2025]. Please always check Government, NHS, local council and other websites for the most up-to-date information, in case there have been changes to these schemes.

Please also note that the author is not a trained medical professional, psychologist, or relationship counsellor. Information shared in this book has been researched and provided based on what helped the author with their own condition(s). However, please note that this should never act as a substitute for consulting your own GP, consultant, mental health/ relationship counselling professional, or healthcare provider first.

Contents

Dedication

For Josh, my rock and soulmate

You inspire me everyday

Acknowledgements

As with many things in life, writing a book is not a solitary endeavour. Whilst the idea, research, and writing have fallen to me, I could not have completed this project without a vast group of people cheering me on behind the scenes.

The biggest thank you goes to my rock and soulmate, Josh. For someone with a way with words, I can't find the words to thank you enough for your ongoing support and belief in me. I feel immensely lucky that you came into my life all those years ago. You have made me feel complete and have enabled me to accomplish my biggest dreams. Huge thanks are due to the other two parts of my dream team, my mum and dad (also known as Linda and Jeff!). You have helped me so much through the rollercoaster ride of being disabled and have given me immense support to achieve my goals and gain my independence. Again, words cannot convey the thanks I owe to you for all you have done throughout my life. I would also like to thank Paul and Carol, my parents-in-law, for their continued support and for bringing my wonderful partner into this world.

I cannot say a big enough thank you to my partner in crime in all things relating to disability equity, the incomparable Johana Hammad. You and I have such a special partnership, and it has been a delight to develop together as co-chairs and close friends over the past few years. Dr Sarah Davison has been another heroine in my story; I cannot quite believe that we have been friends for a decade! Thank you for your guidance and expertise throughout this entire process. You are the kindest friend and the best mother. I would like to thank Jordan Hillier next, for his continued support of our family and for his endless design inspirations. Thank you also to Marek Bielawski and Phoenix Broxton for our friendship and for listening to me ramble about book ideas, research, and writing for the past months. To Johana, Sarah, Jordan, Marek, and Phoenix, thank you for being my squad of cheerleaders.

I could not have undertaken writing this book without the vital support of everyone at the University of Salford. To Team TOFS especially (Alex, Lorraine, Rachel, Marie, Jen P, Fiona, Daisy, Cathy, Jen D, Hannah, and Lesley), you are simply the best, kindest, and most supportive team that anyone could hope for. Thank you for always being there for me, even on my hardest high-pain days, and especially through my recent life-threatening experience. It inspired me so much to know that I am surrounded by your love. I would also like to thank Lord Keith Bradley and Baroness Tanni Grey-Thompson for their continued support of my work, for which I am eternally grateful. My writing has further been shaped by my close working relationship with Professor Simone Buitendijk; Simone, thank you for believing in me and encouraging me in my path to becoming a published author. And to the Access Salford disabled, chronic illness, and neurodivergent staff network at the university, thank you for being a source of inspiration for me, and for supporting me as your co-chair. It is for our community that I wrote this book.

I must extend a considerable thank you to the team at Western Publishing House. You have supported me through every stage of the journey, believed in my vision, and brought it to life. I am so grateful for your expertise and professionalism, and for your help in making *Rolling with It* a reality.

And, finally, thank you to my furry family, past and present—Bruno, Evie, Remy, Snow, Belle, Sylvie, Wakeley, and Ned. With your unconditional love, you have helped me through my hardest days.

About the Author

Dr Lucy Neat-Ward is an up-and-coming author. *Rolling With It: A Guide to Living and Thriving with a Disability* is her debut work. Lucy is both an accomplished writer and public speaker, having published her doctoral thesis in 2022. She has presented talks on disability rights and equity issues on both a national and international scale. She is also an active member of the Disabled Leaders Network and has presented alongside renowned disability advocates on topics including grassroots advocacy. Lucy is a core member of disabled people's organisations locally and nationally in the UK and is dedicated to supporting the disabled community through her writing and advocacy work.

Foreword

If there were ever a time for a book on improving the understanding of the lived experience of Disability, it is now. Disability, a protected characteristic in the UK, is complex and multi-faceted, though significantly under-researched and poorly understood. And yet it reflects one of the largest minoritised groups.

In *Rolling with It*, Lucy May Neat-Ward offers a powerful, practical, and deeply personal guide to navigating life with a Disability in the UK. This book is not only a lifeline for Disabled readers, it is also a vital resource for those of us working in Equality, Diversity, and Inclusion (EDI) spaces, whether or not we choose to identify as Disabled ourselves, and whether or not we choose to share our Disability with others.

Having spent a career at the intersection of statistical education and inclusive practices, I have direct knowledge and lived experience of how often Disabled voices are marginalised in data, policy, and practice. And yet education, and society generally, stand to gain significantly from creating inclusive and accessible places and experiences. This book sets out to achieve this by foregrounding the lived experience of being Disabled while simultaneously offering clear, actionable advice.

Each of the ten chapters is a comprehensive, practical, and empathetic guide for Disabled people in the UK, written by and for the Disability community. Each chapter addresses a different aspect of living and thriving with a Disability, from navigating grief and identity to accessing education, employment, and benefits. The inclusion of reflection prompts at the end of each chapter makes it ideal for personal growth, peer support, and professional development.

Perhaps the most powerful contribution this book makes is in its framing of Disability not as a deficit, but as a journey. Lucy introduces readers to the social model of Disability, which shifts the focus from individual impairment to societal barriers, contrasting this with the medical model. This provides a critical lens for anyone working in Equality, Diversity and Inclusion (EDI) spaces. It reminds us that inclusion is not about fixing people. Rather it is about challenging and fixing systems and barriers. Lucy's writing challenges ableism, medical gaslighting, and the myth of independence. Instead, she celebrates interdependence, community, and Disability pride.

For non-Disabled allies, this book is an invitation to listen, learn, and act. It offers practical guidance on how to support Disabled colleagues, friends, and loved ones, without pity or assumptions. Lucy reminds us that Disability is not a niche issue, and that it is the only marginalised identity group that anyone can join at any time. We are all, in a sense, pre-Disabled. The reality that one day you, too, reader, might be Disabled and that you will be interacting with

Disabled people already – perhaps not even knowingly – calls for compassion, preparation, and solidarity.

Rolling with It will challenge you to think differently. Whether you are Disabled, an ally, a policymaker, or an educator, this book is for you. It offers up tools to assist you and others to advocate for change, to build inclusive environments, and to honour the full spectrum of human experience.

I am proud to support this book and hope it finds its way into classrooms and boardrooms across the country because it's a book that will start the conversation that is so badly needed to create a more Disability inclusive society.

-Jackie

Professor Jackie Carter

Academic Lead: Disability Inclusion, The University of Manchester

Let's start at the beginning...

Disability is rather a bizarre thing when you think about it. Around 20% of the UK population has a disability of some description; some of us are part of this minority from birth, whereas others develop or acquire disabilities throughout their lives. In truth, disability is the only marginalised group that anyone can join at any time. There is also the argument that disability inevitably comes with age, so we are all 'pre-disabled' until we eventually become disabled if we live long enough. At the same time, disability is the most diverse minority in several ways. Not only are there so many different disabilities, but people with the same diagnosis can even experience their disability in vastly different ways or have very different access needs. So yes, disability is a funny old thing that's just part of the great variety that is human life.

However, for the largest marginalised group that anyone might join, there is often the assumption among non-disabled people that our society would put support and accommodations in place to allow us all to access the things we need. Sadly, this couldn't be further from the truth. Despite the gains of the disability rights movement, we continue to live in a largely inaccessible world where it is immensely difficult to access support for disability, where stigma and disability discrimination persist, and where living with a disability comes with a monumental price tag of an additional

£1,000+ per month to have the same quality of life as non-disabled people.[1] The question of disability welfare is highly politically charged in the UK at present, especially following the Labour government's announced plans to cut disability welfare support in the hopes of encouraging disabled people back to work, while there are also plans to reduce some elements of Access to Work support. Despite their professed aims, those in power are not working with employers to educate them about disability, nor are they making more inclusive and accessible jobs available across the UK. It is absurd, too, that political decisions affecting disabled people and their livelihoods are largely made by non-disabled ministers, such is the structure of our society and political system.

In this difficult time for disabled people, we are searching for support more than ever, especially as living with a disability doesn't come with a manual at the best of times. This is what inspired me most to write this book. It is a guide to living and thriving as a disabled person in the UK, written *for* the disability community and *by* a disabled woman. I was born with classical Ehlers-Danlos Syndrome, which began to seriously affect me around the age of seventeen; I was instantly launched into the world of disability, thrown into the deep end without water wings to keep me afloat. I felt completely lost in this strange new world, which I did not know

---

[1] Scope. (2025) Disability Price Tag 2025 [Online]. Available at https://www.scope.org.uk/campaigns/disability-price-tag (Accessed 8 August 2025).

14

how to navigate. At the time, I was also grieving both the life I had already lost and the future life I had envisaged for myself without disability. Some days, I didn't know how to go on and it severely impacted my mental health. I desperately wanted someone to take me by the hand and show me a way through this confusion, to show me that it would be alright, and that life would seem worth living again.

This is where I hope that this book comes in. It is a collection of everything I've learned over the past decade and a half of living, studying, and working with a disability and being immersed in the disabled community, with the hope that it will guide you on your own journey. This is why each chapter ends with a concise 'what I learned' section, to summarise the main takeaways for the topic at hand. I have included some of my own stories in this book, too, as I think that, as disabled people, we often go through shared experiences; I would never want anyone to feel that they were facing it all alone, the way I felt when first dealing with all this at the tender age of seventeen.

So, I hope you'll join me as we explore the next ten chapters together and look at how to thrive with a disability. In the first few chapters, we'll look at adapting to life with a disability, dealing with feelings of grief, and choosing whether to accept your identity as a disabled person. We'll then move on to look at your hobbies and relationships with your friends, family, and potential romantic partner(s). These chapters will explore how to adapt your hobbies and interests around your disability, as well as trying new ones. They'll consider how your relationships may change, and how to find and stay in love when you're disabled. The following chapter will then explore working and studying with a disability in the UK, including the support that is available to you. We'll then look at how to advocate for yourself and how to deal with ableism or discrimination. In the next few chapters, we'll work on pacing your activity levels and protecting your mental and physical health and wellbeing. The final chapters will discuss how you can access mobility aids and give you some top tips for getting around and claiming your independence as a disabled person.

Throughout these chapters, you will see that disability inevitably comes with challenges and curve balls that get thrown your way, and that life as a disabled person can be highly unpredictable. However, I hope that this book will show you that you just need to roll with it (pun absolutely intended for wheelchair users!). My disability has taught me to take life as it comes, roll with the punches to overcome the obstacles, but focus on what you want to achieve in life and find joy in the small moments. The chapters have been carefully considered and ordered to flow in a way that will help you to (re-)build your life and flourish with a disability, if read in sequence. But they also work as stand-alone chapters, so that you can dip in and out as and when you need some support with one of the chapter themes, depending on what your priorities are. So, I hope you'll join me in my wheelchair along for the (st)roll, and I would like to wish you all the best in not just surviving but thriving with your disability.

Chapter 1
So, You're Disabled – Now What?
Adapting to your life with a Disability

So, you've developed or been diagnosed with a disability. Your life may have drastically changed and be unrecognisable from what it once was. You might be asking, What now? How am I supposed to carry on like this? As a society, we have some idea of what to expect with big life changes like getting married, buying a house, or having children. But there's rarely a frame of reference for the huge life upheaval that it can be to become disabled or receive a life-altering diagnosis. It's something we rarely talk about, as if even mentioning disability is still somehow taboo.

Whether you are born with a disability or whether you acquire one later in your life, you will need to learn how to adapt to the world around you. As a disabled person, the world we currently live in is rarely designed with us in mind; it is largely inaccessible, and discrimination linked to disability sadly persists. This nature of our society can make for challenging experiences that – with time – you can learn how to navigate. Acquiring a disability can also generate difficult emotions for you. Particularly if you become disabled later in life or have a progressive condition, you may experience strong feelings about the considerable changes to your life. You're learning to adapt to life with a (worsening) disability, and you might equally be dealing with feelings about the able-bodied life you left behind or the image of what your life could have been without disability in the picture. The remainder of this book will guide you through the practicalities of adapting to – and making the most out of – your life with a disability. Before we dive in, though, I would like to pause here and give some space to the tremendous emotional impact that acquiring a disability can have for some.

It's ok to grieve

A common experience which disabled people often share at the start of their journeys is a feeling of grief. They may grieve the life they had prior to becoming disabled or their condition worsening. They might instead grieve the life that they could have had without their disability. This grief can express itself differently for each person. For some, it may give rise to feelings of extreme sadness or even depression. Others may experience anxiety, anger, or they may even feel like they are numb and apathetic to life going on around them. However you experience this grief, these feelings are completely natural, and it is ok if you experience them on your journey with disability. Try to be gentle with yourself instead and let the feelings flow through you as they arise.

As many people are aware, time is indeed a great healer for grief. Especially as you refocus on the things that matter most to you in your life as a disabled person, you will hopefully realise that you can still lead a full and fulfilling life. However, if you are still struggling

19

with grief or anger, there are some things you can try that might help. Take care of yourself and be kind and gentle to yourself as you grieve; ensure that you eat well, drink plenty of water, get enough sleep, and incorporate gentle movement to support both your body and your mind. Allow your emotions to flow through you, both positive and negative, without judgement. Note them as they pass through you but try not to let them linger. Be patient with yourself, too. Grief can be such a tough experience, and you will have better and worse days. Remember that it is a process, and one that involves different emotions for each of us. There is no timeline to grief, as we all grieve at different speeds. Try not to compare or put pressure on yourself to feel a certain way by a particular point in time.

If you're still struggling with grief, reaching out to close friends or loved ones around you is always a great idea. Explain to them how you're feeling and what kind of support you need; you may just want someone to be a sympathetic ear, but if there is something specific that they can do to help you, tell them exactly what support you need. If you'd rather not talk to those you know, you could consider professional grief counselling instead. This support might help you to navigate the grieving process and to reframe what you are going through. Most of all, though, be compassionate and kind to yourself; you have undergone a major life change, and it will naturally take time to adjust.

Developing new skills from your disability

As time progresses and you recover from grief, you might even find that your disability offers opportunities for personal growth and to broaden your skillset. Navigating life with a disability can be tricky at times, but there are many skills you can develop by rolling with it and working to overcome these barriers. To name but a few:

- **Empathy**: the ability to share and understand others' feelings. As you face your own struggles and emotions relating to your disability, you might cultivate a deeper understanding of the difficulties that other people face and how this can make them feel. You may even share some of the same emotions and so gain the ability to better empathise with others.

- **Emotional intelligence:** being aware of, controlling, and expressing your emotions, whilst handling interpersonal relationships empathetically. As you pass through grief to other emotions, you have the perfect opportunity to learn how to identify, manage, and express your emotions in a more constructive way. Your increasing empathy may help you to navigate your relationships in a more emotionally intelligent way too.

- **Communication:** the ability to convey your ideas and feelings effectively. Being disabled offers many opportunities to practice your communication skills. You may need to reach out and connect to others – whether family and friends, or professional counsellors – to discuss how you're feeling. Talking about your emotions can feel uncomfortable at first, and you may find it difficult to identify how you are feeling. But as your emotional intelligence grows, and as you practice talking about your feelings more, you will find that this becomes easier. Communication skills go together with assertiveness and self-advocacy too (more on this below and in chapter seven). As you learn what your access needs are, practice communicating these to others. The more effectively you can communicate what you need, the more likely it will be that others will be able to understand and help you.

• **Patience:** accepting delays and problems without becoming annoyed or anxious. Being disabled can be extremely frustrating at times, especially when you are faced with inaccessibility, stigma, and ignorant attitudes. It can often take a long time to overcome access barriers, such as waiting for benefit reviews or support at work. This is an excellent opportunity to learn how to patiently accept issues or delays, though you should still persevere until your needs are met!

• **Tenacity:** the determination to continue what you are doing, even when things get tough. Disability certainly teaches you tenacity! This will help you to persevere in the face of adversity, such as when you encounter obstacles to your access needs being met. Sometimes you just have to keep rolling with it and trying different things until you land on a solution.

• **Assertiveness:** being confident when asking for something you need or stating what you believe. When you have a disability, chronic illness, or are neurodivergent, you might find yourself in situations where you will need to stand up for yourself and assert what you need, such as your access requirements. These situations can teach you how to be assertive and how to ask for things so that others respect your requests. You may find it difficult to be assertive at first, but the more you practice, the easier it will feel.

- **Self-advocacy:** the ability to speak up for yourself and communicate your needs to achieve a goal. Together with assertiveness, being disabled will give rise to plenty of occasions where you'll need to advocate for yourself. As you learn more about your disability, you will gain a greater understanding of what your access needs are. Due to inaccessibility and ableism, there will undoubtedly be instances where you must self-advocate, such as gaining access to venues and events or even getting support in your workplace. Again, this skill may not come naturally at first, but the more you practice, the more second-nature it will become to you.

- **Adaptability and flexibility:** adjusting to new and unfamiliar conditions. Given the inaccessible nature of our world, there will be times when you will need to be flexible to achieve your goals. For instance, if you are a wheelchair user, you might research a route to a job interview which you believe to be accessible to you. However, when you discover that this route is littered with cobblestones, you will need to adapt to still get to that interview. You may in the future learn how to wheelie over bumpy terrain such as cobblestones, affording you greater independence. As you experience more and more of these situations, you will know better how to adapt to ensure that you can still achieve your goals with a disability – it is a skill which comes with time and experience.

• **Creativity:** using your imagination or coming up with original ideas to make something new. Especially when you face barriers, being disabled can lead to opportunities for you to think more creatively. For example, if you are blind or partially sighted, you may have difficulty telling apart different eye shadow palettes which all feel the same. To resolve this, you may come up with the idea to use tactile stick-on gems to create different patterns or braille on each palette to tell them apart, or research how to use a braille labeller. Sometimes, when faced with obstacles to enjoying your life, you will need to think creatively about the problem to find a practicable solution.

• **Organisational skills:** being efficient and systematic in managing your time, energy, and resources. These skills can support you in meeting deadlines, planning your workload, setting goals, and delegating tasks where needed. Being disabled can allow you to develop strong organisational skills. Say you wish to go on a day out with friends, but you are an assistance-dog handler with other access needs. Sadly, it's no longer as simple as just turning up on the day. You may need to research which venues are accessible for you and suitable for your dog, and so you might have to call to ask for access information. You will also need to plan what items your dog needs for the duration of the day, as well as planning your route and allocating additional time in case of travel delays. When you're

24

disabled, a lot of planning and organisation can go into the smallest of things. Given the barriers and challenges that can come with being disabled, there are plenty of occasions to really hone your organisational skills.

• **Acceptance:** the willingness to tolerate a difficult situation. Whilst at first you may experience feelings of grief and anger related to your disability, with time, these feelings do tend to fade. Many people do eventually accept their disability as part of their identity and lived experience. The path to acceptance may be hard for you, but it is worth it to feel a sense of peace with your life and who you are. As you open yourself up to different ways of thinking about disability – such as the social model that we'll cover in chapter two – you might come to accept that your disability itself is not a barrier; the issue is that we currently live in a society that is still largely inaccessible for many disabled people. Acceptance comes in different forms, but it is a vital quality to cultivate if you want to thrive with a disability!

Adapting to becoming disabled, then, does not just entail anger and grief, but is far more multifaceted than that. There are many skills that being disabled gives you the opportunity to cultivate, and many ways to grow as a person, if you remain open to the possibilities.

My experience

When my disability first became severe around the age of seventeen, I went through a lot of emotions as things progressed. At first, I was angry that I was no longer able to do things as easily as my peers or do things that they took for granted, like showering easily or getting to college independently. When I then went off to university, I continued to become increasingly ill to the point that most of my Fresher's week and the first few weeks of my university life – when I should have been enjoying my new-found freedom and Fresher life – were spent in and out of hospitals. When it became clear that this illness was not something easy to diagnose or treat (indeed, after a misdiagnosis, it took another 7 years to be diagnosed with classical Ehlers-Danlos Syndrome) and that it would be long-term, I took the difficult decision to interrupt my studies and come home for a year of medical tests and treatment.

On the day that I left my first university, I so clearly remember sitting on my window ledge seat in my student room with hot, silent tears streaming down my face. Quite simply, I was grieving. I experienced an intense feeling of loss, not just for the university place I had given up, but for the future that I had dreamt of for myself ever since being a little girl. It all felt impossibly out of reach, and I couldn't picture how on earth I was meant to go on. The silent tears of grief continued throughout the three-hour car ride home with my dad, and for days and weeks after I had settled back into life at home.

With time, the grief thankfully began to pass. It no longer felt like a hot knife that had been plunged into my chest. Instead, this feeling was replaced by a numbness and an apathy. Without any clear direction in my life, it was hard to muster any motivation or set goals that I wanted to achieve. But as the year passed, and we made some progress on the medical front, I became more used to the idea of living my life as a disabled woman. The anger and the grief largely passed, and I even began to dream again of what my future could be, although the vision was very different from the non-disabled life that I had held on to for so many years.

Despite this more positive outlook, I still had good days and bad days. Sometimes, the challenges that came with being disabled wore me down, making me cry frustrated tears and threaten to give up. As my mum and boyfriend would frequently remind me, though, giving up was not an option. Anyone who knows me well – and especially my husband – will tell you that I am a *very* stubborn person. Spurred on by my support team, I was determined to face these obstacles head-on and to just roll with whatever came my way. I began to change the way I thought about the challenges that came with disability, seeing them instead as opportunities to grow as a person and to develop new skills. I learned a lot along the way as I faced these challenges, becoming a more resilient and confident person.

Later in my life, adapting to becoming a manual wheelchair user certainly presented me with some challenges, but also the opportunity to develop many of the qualities we discussed above.

When we purchased our first home – a house that wasn't fully accessible, but which had so much potential – I couldn't navigate my wheelchair over the steep lipped steps of the front or back doors. As I had lived with my disability for a few years by this point, I knew that I needed a wheelchair-accessible way of entering and exiting our home and back garden more easily if I was to be able to get around independently.

By this point, I was somewhat used to self-advocacy and asserting my access needs, but this was on a new scale. Never had I been to a council to advocate for myself. By using the skills that I had already honed by dealing with other obstacles, I was assertive and communicated effectively to ask them to assist with building ramps into our property. Unfortunately, the council informed me that the terrain around our home just wasn't suitable to construct the kind of ramps they offered. But they *could* offer some shallow graded steps to be built in our back garden. Now was the time for tenacity! Thinking creatively about the problem, I realised I could use some of the wheelchair skills I had been practising to surmount the shallow graded steps. I asked the council to install the steps, then spent hours watching videos of how to pop a little wheelie and then practised endlessly in my living room with the help of soft sofas and rugs to fall back on! By the time the council had fully installed our new steps, I was a pro at popping wheelies and could easily climb the steps in my wheelchair.

However, I still had the problem of how I was to enter our front door. Again, I took inspiration from things I had seen from other disabled people on social media, and I roughly designed a wooden ramp that could be made with decking materials to make our front door more accessible to me. I then approached a family member who was particularly skilled at woodworking to discuss the possibility of building the ramp. Our relative kindly agreed and so I waited for the ramp to be constructed and eventually fitted to our front door. After its installation, I cautiously tested it to see if I could successfully access our door and … I'm pleased to say, mission accomplished!

I hope that this story shows that it's natural to have different emotions after you've become disabled, as it is a truly life changing moment. Don't rush your emotions; just roll with them and let them flow through you at their own pace, as time is often a great healer. Alternatively, you could challenge your way of thinking and reframe the difficult emotions and obstacles that come with being disabled as opportunities for growth. As my story of adapting to becoming a wheelchair-user shows – from just one experience related to my disability – came the opportunity to grow several skills and qualities that later would help me to navigate life. I advocated for myself, I was assertive, I communicated effectively, I was tenacious, I thought creatively, used organisational skills, and practiced patience. All these skills I honed thanks to my disability!

So, how do you ultimately adapt to becoming disabled?

Adapting to a disability may come with feelings of grief and anger, although it's perfectly natural and ok to grieve or to feel a loss. After all, your life has undergone a massive change! But becoming disabled is about so much more than grief and loss. It can expand your horizons, it allows you to hone various skills, and it encourages personal growth, if you give it the chance. I'd even say that adapting to becoming disabled made me a better and more empathetic person. Having a disability also means a life of constant change and adaptation as your condition changes. As we'll see in the next chapter, disability is far from static. It is fluid and changeable, and something you learn to roll with and grow alongside.

What I learned:

- It's ok to grieve when you acquire or are diagnosed with a disability. Be kind to yourself, you've just undergone a major life change.

- There are a lot of things that you can learn from being disabled, if you're open to it. Don't close yourself off to the possibilities that come with life with a disability.

- It may take time, but you will see that being disabled is about more than grief and loss. You have so much to look forward to in this life.

Reflection Time:

1. Do you feel any grief related to your disability? If so, can you pinpoint exactly what is causing your grief? Identifying these emotions is the first step in addressing them.

2. How do you think your disability might help you to develop as a person? Are there any skills that you are eager to learn in particular?

3. Following your answer to question (2), think about how you might go about developing these skills and jot down your ideas.

Chapter 2
Becoming a Proud Disabled Woman
Regaining your identity and self-confidence

In the last chapter, we looked at how to adapt to becoming disabled, including acceptance. Many people do with time come to accept their disability as a central part of their life and sometimes even as a part of their identity. However, becoming disabled can affect your self-confidence, especially if your life and body have gone through sudden changes. This chapter will look at how we understand disability and how it can come to shape our identity as disabled people. We will consider how your disability might inform your identity, as well as how accepting your disability can lead to you regaining and even growing in self-confidence.

To be, or not to be disabled, that is the question!

Before we look at different ways of thinking about disability, how stereotypes can damage our self-esteem, and how to regain your self-confidence, I feel that a few words on identity are warranted. Over time, I have come to accept my disability as a key part of my identity, as it impacts pretty much every life experience that I have and shapes my interactions with the world. I'm therefore a proud disabled woman.

Whilst many disabled people do come to accept their disability as part of their identity, there is absolutely no rule or pressure to say that you *must* do this. Our identities are highly personal, and you have a choice over whether you wish to identify as disabled or not. Even within the disabled community, we all identify differently. For instance, some people with chronic illnesses do not identify as 'disabled' but prefer to refer to themselves as a 'spoonie' or someone with a chronic illness. Similarly, those in the d/Deaf community tend not to consider themselves disabled at all. It's completely up to you how you identify; choose what feels best for you in the moment, and remember that our identities are not static, but may change over time.

Although our identities are fluid and changeable, as an author, I need some way of referring to disability which covers as many potential readers as possible. Within this book, then, whenever you read 'disabled', know that this encompasses anyone with a physical or mental health condition, those with chronic or 'non-apparent' illnesses, those who are neurodivergent, those who are blind or partially sighted, those who are d/Deaf or hard of hearing, those with learning disabilities, and anyone else who self-identifies as 'disabled'. I have tried to be as inclusive as possible, but if I've accidentally missed anyone out, please know that you are welcome here! Now that we've cleared that up, let's move on to consider what even is a disability?!

What is a disability?

Ok, I know that this question might seem a bit of a bizarre one in a book about how to thrive as a disabled person. You might think the answer is obvious, a complete no-brainer. But please bear with me, as disability is a fluid concept and there are various ways to understand what it is. Let's start with the legal definition in the UK. Under the Equality Act 2010, a disability is a 'physical or mental impairment that has a substantial and negative long-term effect on your ability to do normal daily activities'.[2] This definition is far from perfect, though, as it remains somewhat medicalised and regards disability as an 'impairment' and something that has a 'negative effect' on our lives. Not all disabled people would agree that this is how they see their disability.

Thankfully, the legal definition is by no means the only way of conceptualising what it is to be disabled. Disability itself is far from static. Instead, you might think of disability as a spectrum which encompasses a diverse range of conditions from learning disabilities to deafness, being a wheelchair user to blindness, or mental health conditions to neurodiversity and more. Even people who share the same disability or diagnosis can have vastly different lived experiences. Crucially, neither our understanding of disability, nor our identities as disabled people, are fixed either. The way that

---

[2] UK Government, (2010) Definition of disability under the Equality Act 2010 [Online]. Available at https://www.gov.uk/definition-of-disability-under-equality-act-2010 (Accessed 8 August 2025).

society perceives disability is constantly evolving. At the start of the disability rights movement in the 1970s, you'd have been hard pressed to convince most people that disabled people belonged in the workplace, in recreational spaces, or even in the media. Nowadays, attitudes have changed dramatically to the extent that most people would now likely agree that disabled people deserve equal opportunities and that non-discriminatory attitudes and reasonable adjustments should be enshrined in law.

The fluidity of disability is also expressed in the idea of a dynamic disability; this means that a person's disability changes in severity, or it might have a different impact upon their life at different times. For example, someone may experience varying levels of chronic pain and fatigue, which affect their mobility differently over time. Some days they might be able to manage walking with crutches, whereas on other days they need to use a wheelchair. Their symptoms and access needs fluctuate according to their periods of remission or flare-ups. They are no more or less disabled just because the severity of their condition fluctuates. Rather, they are dynamically disabled.

Finally, disability may fluctuate between being visible and being non-apparent. Non-apparent disabilities are physical, mental, or neurological conditions which are not immediately evident just from looking at someone from the outside. These conditions might include chronic fatigue or pain, mental health conditions, learning disabilities, or ADHD and autism. At times, though, these disabilities may be more apparent than at others, such as if you're using an aid like a walking stick, a fidget device, or noise-cancelling headphones to support you. Some dislike the label 'invisible disabilities', as they argue that there are always ways to infer someone's disability, if you are paying close enough attention; this is why I have used the term non-apparent disability in this book.

Overall, the nature of disability is constantly evolving. Excitingly, this can mean that our identities as disabled people are open to change, especially if we accept our disability as a core part of our identity. In addition to this flexibility, though, there are several other factors which might shape how we see ourselves and our disability. Let's look at a few.

The social and medical models of disability

One thing which can alter the way we perceive our disability is by considering it through the lens of either the social or medical model of disability. Let me explain. The medical model has by far been the prominent way of thinking about disability historically. It sees disability as a problem within the disabled person and so focuses on diagnosing and treating their medical condition. But the medical model does not consider society's role in creating discriminatory and ableist attitudes around disability, nor the way in which our society erects barriers and makes things inaccessible for disabled people. The medical model equally reinforces the idea that medical professionals must intervene and 'improve' disabled people's lives.

On a more positive note, though, this model has led to medical breakthroughs, some of which have considerably improved the lives of disabled people and given them greater independence. For example, implanted in my back, I have a sacral nerve modulator which stimulates the nerves needed to urinate; it thereby reduces my reliance on catheters and affords me more independence. On the other hand, though, the medical model is deeply problematic as a way of thinking about disability. It essentially regards disabled people as something to be 'fixed' or 'cured', which is an ableist narrative that devalues our personhood. Ableism is discrimination in favour of non-disabled people, and in an ableist society it's assumed that the 'normal' way to live is as a non-disabled person. The medical model is intertwined with ableism, as it regards disabled bodies and minds as defective and less valuable compared to non-disabled people. It creates low expectations for and of disabled people, and leads to them losing independence, control, and choice over their lives.

This is where the social model of disability intervenes, and it has increasingly been gaining traction with the rise of the disability rights movement since the 1970s. This model considers disability to be a social issue created by society's predominant practices, rather than thinking that there is something inherently 'wrong' with disabled people. Instead, it is society's lack of access and its

37

discriminatory attitudes towards disabled people which end up disabling them. The social model consequently seeks to remove barriers which restrict life choices and independence for disabled people. It calls for the need to create policies which promote inclusion and accessibility on a wider scale. Perhaps most importantly, the social model was itself devised by disabled people as they felt that the medical model did not account for their lived experiences of disability, nor did it foster more inclusive practices and ways of living.

Let's take a few examples to highlight the differences between the medical and social models of disability. Think of a wheelchair user who is paralysed from a spinal cord injury. According to the medical model, they are disabled by the injury to their spinal cord which paralyses them, and the inability of current medical science to cure this condition. They are disabled as there is something perceived to be at fault in their body. By contrast, according to the social model, the wheelchair user is disabled because society remains largely inaccessible to them; building ramps or ensuring that venues are wheelchair accessible is currently the exception, rather than standard practice. The wheelchair user is essentially disabled as the world around them isn't set up in a way that is inclusive of their access needs.

Let's think now of a blind or partially sighted person. If we take the medical model, this person is disabled by a medical condition affecting their eyesight - such as glaucoma, retinitis pigmentosa or incontinentia pigmenti – and which cannot currently be cured by medical interventions. According to the social model instead, they are disabled because society by and large does not accommodate their access needs. This is due to the lack of information available in braille, large print, audio, or alternative formats, the lack of tactile paving on pavements, or websites not being accessible for screen readers. The blind or partially sighted person is further disabled due to persistent discriminatory and ableist attitudes towards their disability.

As you can see, the medical and social models can greatly alter how we perceive disability. For disabled people, these models can have a very tangible impact on our confidence and self-esteem. For years, I had been conditioned by the society I had grown up in to perceive disability through the medical model. When I was then diagnosed with a genetic disease in my mid-twenties, I strongly believed that there was something 'wrong' with me and my body due to having faulty collagen, and something that I clearly wasn't trying hard enough to fix as I was just getting worse and worse. I even began to blame myself for developing my disability, when it was really all down to my genetics – something I had very little say over (p.s. thanks mum and dad)! When I finally learnt about the social model of disability a few years later, it felt like a fog was lifting and I could now see the light. It started a slow process of reconstructing a more positive relationship with my disabled body and rebuilding my lost self-confidence. It also gave me a focal point that I could work towards changing; I couldn't change my genetics, but I could work hard to influence society's attitudes towards disability and fight for my access needs to be met.

The social model can be transformative in how we think about our disabilities and how they shape our identity. It no longer puts the onus on us as disabled people, nor does it insist that there is something defective about us. It instead looks to society to be more inclusive and accepting. But the medical and social models only account for two ways of perceiving disability. There are other factors, including disability stereotypes, which can also influence how we see ourselves and our disabilities.

Disability stereotypes

Disability stereotypes continue to be prevalent in our society; whilst some can be uplifting and life-changing in how they help us to reframe disability, others can be ableist and incredibly damaging for disabled people. Every Paralympic year, we all know the stereotypes well. Paralympians are physically and metaphorically put on pedestals and are lauded as inspirational heroes and heroines for overcoming the odds to achieve excellence in their chosen sport. Now, don't get me wrong – the achievements of elite athletes at the pinnacle of their sport are amazing, and they deserve to be celebrated for their incredible sporting achievements. But, in contrast to their Olympic counterparts, Paralympians are often built up as inspirations for *overcoming* their disability to succeed in sport.

Their disability, then, is considered as something that will hinder them and that must be conquered, rather than as something that is intrinsic to who they are.

These stereotypical representations of disabled people in the public consciousness tend to reflect contemporaneous ideas in science, medicine, religion, and social discourse, including the medical model of disability. But why do we construct these stereotypes? Well, stereotypes often arise from an urge to categorise the world around us, to make it easier for us to comprehend. The issue is that this approach can lead us to over-simplify a diverse subset of people and create potentially harmful stereotypes, which often operate at extreme ends of the spectrum of disability. Disabled people are either viewed as Paralympic heroes and inspirations, or benefit scroungers who cannot or do not want to work, and who are consequently a drain on our welfare resources.

With harmful stereotypes, though, the good thing is that we can do some myth-busting to resist them. Let's look at a few pervasive stereotypes about disability and how we can challenge them. One stereotype holds that all disabled people are brave and courageous for overcoming the hardships that our disabilities can pose. Adapting to new life circumstances may indeed mean that there are challenges and obstacles to overcome, which may call for courage and bravery. However, non-disabled people should be careful not to turn our lived experiences of disability into inspiration porn; this is the objectification of disabled people for the benefit of non-disabled people. Praising disabled people disproportionately for 'overcoming' the perceived difficulties associated with their disability and pigeon-holing them into being inspirational figures falls right into this trope. It over-simplifies our lived experiences of disability, and does not allow us to be full, rounded individuals with our own unique experiences, skills, desires, and interests. Allowing us to live as our multi-faceted and complex selves gives a much more accurate representation of the disabled experience than any stereotype ever could.

Another ubiquitous stereotype is that disabled people are benefit scroungers who do not wish to work or who are 'faking it', and who are thus a drain on the welfare system. This is once again an over-simplification of lived disabled experience. Whilst disabled people may sometimes need to get support from the welfare system, this is rarely because they do not *want* to work. Rather, employment is not made accessible to disabled people, and so they are excluded from certain – often higher earning – positions. The idea that they might be 'faking' having a disability or health condition just to receive benefits is also erroneous. Recent studies have shown that the fraud rate for benefits like Personal Independence Payment is currently around 0%.[3] There is a genuine need for welfare support for disabled

---

[3] UK Government. (16 May 2024) Fraud and error in the benefit system, Financial Year Ending (FYE) 2024 [Online]. Available at https://www.gov.uk/government/statistics/fraud-and-error-in-the-benefit-system-financial-year-2023-to-2024-estimates/fraud-and-error-in-the-benefit-system-

people. Research by disability charity Scope has recently shown that it costs on average about £1,010 per month more for a disabled person to have the same standard of living as a non-disabled person in the UK.[4] Whilst this stereotype clearly does not hold true, it can still be extremely damaging for disabled people. It draws them into a heated social and political dialogue about the welfare state and the allocation of benefits and so can inspire hatred and even hate crimes towards them.

A final widespread stereotype is that it is too costly for companies to make reasonable adjustments for employees with disabilities to enable them to work safely. This perceived cost is sometimes used as a reason to deny adjustments to disabled colleagues, further contributing to their reliance on the welfare system. Yet the truth is that most reasonable adjustments only come with minimal cost to the employer. Research by Deloitte shows that 57% of employees with disabilities do not need additional accommodations;[5] for those that do, research by the Business Disability Forum shows that the average cost is only around £75 per

financial-year-ending-fye-2024#personal-independence-payment-overpayments-and-underpayments (Accessed 8 August 2025).

[4] Scope. (2025) Disability Price Tag 2025 [Online]. Available at https://www.scope.org.uk/campaigns/disability-price-tag (Accessed 8 August 2025).

[5] Deloitte. (2024) Deloitte's first Disability Inclusion @ Work 2024 survey reveals that workplace accessibility is a significant challenge for many [Online]. Available at https://www.deloitte.com/global/en/about/press-room/deloittes-first-disability-inclusion-work-2024.html (Accessed 8 August 2025).

person.[6] Although not true, then, this stereotype is nevertheless extremely damaging to disabled people, to the extent of completely excluding them from employment.

Ableist stereotypes about disability rarely hold true, then. But they can still impact on how we see ourselves as disabled people, especially if we internalise such ableist stereotypes. So-called internalised ableism is when a disabled person absorbs and acts on negative beliefs and prejudices about disability which are prevalent within society. It can lead to them rejecting their disabled identity to instead align with ableist 'norms'. Such internalised ableism and ableist stereotypes are further damaging as they can lower your self-confidence and self-esteem. It might make you feel like you do not belong in the disabled community, that you are not 'disabled enough', or that you do not deserve reasonable adjustments. It might also lead you to compare yourself too much to non-disabled or neurotypical people, and to then place unrealistic expectations on yourself. Over time, ableist stereotypes and internalised ableism can slowly chip away at your self-confidence until there is barely anything left.

---

[6] Business Disability Forum. (11 September 2024) Reasonable adjustments – what are they and why are they important [Online]. Available at https://businessdisabilityforum.org.uk/resource/reasonable-adjustments-smes/ (Accessed 8 August 2025).

When I was twenty-one years old and at university, I experienced the harmful nature of ableist stereotypes and internalism ableism. I could sometimes walk on crutches at the time, and on many occasions, I was accused of being a benefit scrounger and faker by people I came across on the street. They would also ask intrusive questions such as what was 'wrong' with me, or even whether I could have sex. Being relatively newly disabled and somewhat fragile, I internalised these messages and it gnawed away at my self-confidence. The internalised ableism led me to place unrealistic expectations on myself to succeed at my work and my studies, to prove I was successful, that there was nothing 'wrong' with me and that I was not a scrounger like others thought. I further convinced myself that I was not 'disabled enough' to use aids like a wheelchair which would have helped me as I increasingly struggled to walk. I isolated myself from the disability community too, as I felt like a fraud in their company for not being 'disabled enough'.

These feelings were not a fleeting phase but persisted for many years throughout my undergraduate degree. The turning point came when a friend finally encouraged me to give social media a try just as I was entering my master's studies. Through the screen of my phone, I soon discovered a thriving and compassionate disability community, with others just like me out there living their truth as proud disabled people. The more people I followed, the more I learnt about internalised ableism, the social model of disability, and how to challenge disability stereotypes. Throughout my master's studies and my time as a PhD researcher, I leant into this online community and felt uplifted by it. My confidence grew and I began to challenge the thoughts that I was not 'disabled enough' or that I was a 'fraud' for being part of the community and for using aids that would help me. Now in my thirties and feeling the most confident in my identity as a proud disabled woman that I've ever been, I so wish I could go back and hug that young woman who was struggling so much. I would tell her how loved she was, how accepted she was just for being her wonderful self, and I would help her to rebuild her self-confidence in the face of ableist stereotypes and internalised ableism.

We have seen just how injurious ableist stereotypes, inspiration porn, and internalised ableism can be, especially given how pervasive they are in our society that we are bombarded with them every day. As these stereotypes can devastate disabled people's self-confidence and self-esteem, what can we do to resist this, to feel self-confident and to accept our disability as part of our identity if we choose to?

Why build confidence in your disabled identity?

An important part of adjusting to life with a disability is accepting it as a core part of your identity, if you wish to do so. But this can be hard to do when faced with pervasive ableist narratives and stereotypes which tell us that our disability is a negative thing. This is why it is crucial to build self-confidence as a disabled person,

46

as it will help you to face challenges and to get back up and try again if you aren't successful the first time. Growing your self-confidence can improve your relationships with others too, as it can help you to communicate effectively and build trust and understanding. Confidence can also support you to be more assertive and to stand up for your rights and access needs, a key skill to self-advocate for yourself as a disabled person. Finally, confidence allows you to express yourself more authentically and to just be yourself, which can lead to positive wellbeing and acceptance of your disabled identity.

How to build your self-confidence

Improving your self-confidence, then, has multiple benefits not only in your personal life as a disabled person, but in the world of work, or in your leisure pursuits, or volunteering. But how might we go about doing this, I hear you ask. Well, there are several things you can do to start cultivating self-confidence today:

- **Stop comparing yourself to others.** With social media showing the highlight reels of everyone's lives these days, it can be hard not to compare yourself and your life to that of others. However, such comparisons are more likely to decrease your self-confidence as you feel envy when you compare yourself, and the more envy we feel, the worse we feel about ourselves. Comparison is truly toxic to our self-confidence, but it's something many of us seem drawn to do and so stopping can be easier said than done. So, how can we go about this? You could remind yourself each day, or whenever you feel the urge to compare yourself, that comparisons aren't helpful. Remember instead that we all have our own lives, achievements, and timeframes which will be right for our lives. Life isn't a competition at the end of the day. It might help you to recount your accomplishments, strengths, and goals. You could consider keeping a gratitude journal in which each day you write down three things for which you are grateful, however big or small (you can find more advice on this in chapter eight). Then, when you feel drawn into making comparisons, you have a record of the wonderful person that you are and your successes, which can help you to refocus on your own journey. Finally, if you feel that social media or other media are encouraging you to compare yourself, you could avoid, mute, or delete these apps.

- **Surround yourself with positivity.** Research has shown that the people with whom you surround yourself can influence your thoughts and attitudes about yourself – in other words, who you make friends with matters to your health and your self-confidence.[7] Surround yourself with

---

[7] National Institutes of Health. (2021) The Power of Peers: Who influences your health [Online]. Available at https://newsinhealth.nih.gov/2021/09/power-

people who are your cheerleaders, who celebrate your successes with you, and who lift you up when you are feeling down or anxious. By seeking out others who have a positive approach to life, you can work on building up your self-confidence. As well as your friends, surround yourself with positivity more broadly. You might introduce daily affirmations into your morning routine to focus your attention on the positive things in your life. You could practice positive self-talk in front of the mirror before your shower or bath. This can include things about yourself that you like or that you're proud of, but it can also help you to approach negative experiences in a more productive and positive way. If you made a mistake at work, for instance, you might say 'making mistakes is human – tomorrow is a fresh chance to try again'. When practiced regularly, positive self-talk promotes self-confidence, lowers stress, and fosters self-compassion to take on new and exciting challenges.

- **Practice self-care.** It's hard to feel good and confident about yourself if you're not looking after your body and mind or even ignoring their needs. You're essentially sending the message to your subconscious that you do not matter. When you believe you matter and look

peers#:~:text=Positive%20and%20negative%20peer%20influences,them%2C%20the%20happier%20you%20are (Accessed 8 August 2025).

after yourself and wellbeing, it builds your confidence as you are doing something positive for yourself. If this is difficult for you, imagine you are talking to a friend – you would naturally tell them that they are important and to take care of themselves, as you care about them. Try to then take your own advice and eat well, drink plenty of water, practice gentle movement, and consider mindfulness or meditative practices. When you care for yourself, you are projecting to the world that you are important, and it builds your self-confidence and self-esteem.

- **Be kind to yourself.** When we're feeling low on self-confidence, we might be tempted to be hard on ourselves and put emphasis on all our mistakes, thereby making ourselves feel worse and even worthless. Instead, practice self-compassion and treat yourself with kindness when you make a mistake or experience a set-back. You could remind yourself that it's natural to make mistakes and that there are often ways to learn from them and create second chances for yourself. You could instead say to yourself that making mistakes actually allows you to develop your emotional intelligence and self-compassion. Research has connected practicing self-compassion with cultivating self-confidence, meaning that being kind and compassionate to yourself is integral to leading a confident life.[8]

- **Face your fears.** Don't wait until you feel more self-confident to face your fears or to tackle a problem. Let's say you're a mobility aid user and you're not feeling confident about going out on your own in case something will be inaccessible to you. If you do not face your fears, you may lose even more confidence and independence and become increasingly isolated if you do not leave the house alone. One of the best ways to build self-confidence in such a situation is to instead face your fear and go out with a friend or on your own; you will likely learn that the reality is not as bad as you had imagined and will build even more confidence each time you go out and things run smoothly. You might also want to do your research before facing your fear, in this case, researching whether venues, roads, and modes of transport are accessible for you and your mobility aids. You can then face your fears with even more confidence, as you are armed with information and prepared for the task at hand. Facing your fears, then, is one of the

---

[8] Positive Psychology. (2 June 2019) How to practice self-compassion: 8 techniques and tips [Online]. Available at https://positivepsychology.com/how-to-practice-self-compassion/#:~:text=Self%2Dcompassion%20involves%20treating%20yourself,routines%20foster%20greater%20self%2Dcompassion. (Accessed 8 August 2025).

best ways to build confidence in situations which are giving you undue stress or anxiety.

- **Know when to say no.** Doing things which you're good at or facing your fears can feel good. For each one of us, though, there are certain things which drain your self-confidence every time that you do them. This is completely natural, and saying no to these activities is incredibly important. For me, singing in front of an audience always makes me feel underconfident and so I am someone who will refuse to give it my all at karaoke. There is absolutely nothing wrong with knowing yourself and your boundaries and keeping to them – in fact, it is a very positive thing indeed! Asserting your boundaries helps to establish a feeling of self-control over your life and can even increase your feelings of self-confidence.

As you work on these steps, you may find that your self-confidence goes from strength to strength, and that you might accept your identity as a disabled person more and more. These processes can take a while, and it is entirely natural for your confidence to build slowly. Acceptance of your identity as a disabled person may develop alongside your self-confidence, or it may be more delayed; it can take a while to accept your disability and your disabled identity, and that's nothing to worry about. We all get there on our own timeframes. Remember that you are on your own unique journey in life, and that you do not need to compare your life to anyone else's.

During my first few years of being disabled, my self-confidence and self-esteem took a big hit. My life had changed so much it was almost unrecognisable. I could no longer do things that I easily managed before, such as going to college or going out with friends, and I now needed to rely on mobility aids to help me get around. As a student just heading off to university and hoping to gain independence, I instead felt reliant on so many aids and people to help to do things for me. I was incredibly self-conscious of my mobility aids, as none of my peers used any. My first mobility aids were clunky, grey, and ugly and so I felt that I stuck out like a sore thumb. My confidence took a further knock when I noticed that my body had begun to change with my disability; my shoulder sunk and looked lop-sided, my spine curved, I put on some weight due to medication side-effects, my fingers were often sore and crooked, and so I dropped things a lot. I had rarely felt confident in my body anyway, but as it changed with my disability, I felt even more ashamed of it. When I later graduated from university with my degree, my confidence was at one of its lowest points in my life.

When it came to getting married shortly after I graduated, my confidence was still at rock bottom. As we prepared for the big day, my fiancé and I built in so many contingencies to hide my disability. We booked a venue with a small side room that would be my sanctuary, where I could take my medications, apply aids, and rest as my body dictated, away from the eyes of our guests. I wore a long dress to hide the knee braces and KT tape holding me together, and I swore off my crutches for the day. My mum was on standby to support me; only moments before I walked down the aisle, she was fixing my knee braces and handing me pain medications to get me through the ceremony. My fiancé insisted that I was perfect as I was and that I should just use my crutches to reduce pain and fatigue on the day, but internalised ableism had well and truly gotten to me. I was convinced that brides had to be visions of perfection, without the trappings of disability revealing how broken I felt that I was. Looking back on it now, I wish that I'd had the confidence to rock my crutches down the aisle and to just be myself on our wedding day. But building confidence in yourself as a disabled person takes time, and I still had a way to go in becoming the bad ass disabled woman I am today.

The journey to regain my confidence was a slow one and took the duration of my doctoral degree and my first few years in full-time employment. There are still days when I need to keep working on it even now. As I crept towards my thirties, I came to realise that my confidence wasn't dependent on having the 'perfect' body (whatever that even is!) or on not using my mobility aids. Instead, I focused on what I *did* have and on what this amazing disabled body of mine had enabled me to achieve. It helped me to complete and be awarded a PhD, to start building a career in full-time employment, to find the energy to engage in wheelchair rugby, and to help co-chair the disability, chronic illness, and neurodivergent colleague network at work, not to mention writing this book whilst recovering in hospital from a pulmonary embolism! As a disabled person, I was out there in the world having an impact and making a difference – and, if you ask me, that's pretty darn amazing. By reducing toxic comparisons, surrounding myself with positivity, and focusing instead of my successes, I slowly built my self-confidence and began to feel proud that I was a strong disabled woman who was thriving. Don't get me wrong, I do still have confidence wobbles when I need my husband and my parents to remind me of what I've achieved. It's natural to wobble. What counts is that we pick ourselves up at the end, carry our self-confidence with us, and come back stronger the next time around.

We've looked at how there are many ways to think about disability and to incorporate your disability into your identity. Some ways of conceptualising disability, such as the social model, are positive and supportive for disabled people, whilst other concepts and stereotypes are less helpful. At the end of the day, it is up to you to decide how you choose to understand disability and whether you do or do not identify as a disabled person; there is no pressure either way. How you identify with your disability might also be closely intertwined with your self-confidence and self-esteem. Acquiring a disability may initially knock your confidence, but as this chapter has shown, there are several ways in which you can intervene and rebuild your self-confidence.

Accepting disability as part of your identity and bolstering your self-confidence are only two small parts of what it means to be a disabled person, though. As humans we are multifaceted beings with many things which make us who we are, and the following chapters will consider some of these different facets of our lives. One important component of who we are comprises our hobbies and interests, so let's take a closer look at adapting these around our disabilities.

What I learned:

- There are many ways to think about disability, and it's ok to choose the one that fits best with how you feel.

- Unfortunately, there are some rather polarised stereotypes that persist around disability; you're either a paralympic hero defying your disability, or a faker and benefit-scrounger. Remember that these ableist stereotypes do not hold true and try not to let them interfere with you living your life as the stunning disabled god or goddess that you are.

- It's ultimately up to you whether you accept your disability as part of your identity. But living and building confidence in this identity can help you to thrive and roll with the challenges that come with being disabled in an ableist and inaccessible world.

- Take the journey to accept your identity and build self-confidence at your own pace and don't beat yourself up if this doesn't happen overnight. We are all unique and amazing individuals on our own journeys and timelines.

Reflection Time

1. What does disability mean to you? How does this impact on how you see yourself and your disability?

2. Do the social and medical models change how you see your disability at all? If so, how?

3. Can you think of any other disability stereotypes? How do they make you feel? How might you challenge these stereotypes?

4. What actions will you take to work on improving your self-confidence?

Chapter 3
Who's up for Murder Ball?

Hobbies and interests

Building your confidence and accepting your identity as a disabled person is only part of what makes you who you are; there is far more to you than just your disability, although this is an important part which shapes your lived experiences. There are many things which make you *you*, including your relationships, your hobbies and interests, or your work or education, and so forth. We'll look at each of these over the next few chapters, starting here with your hobbies and interests.

We're all passionate about different things, and there is rarely just *one* thing which captures our interest. Your hobbies and interests can help you to build self-confidence and reinforce positive aspects of your personality, such as leadership, collaboration, and compassion, as well as boosting our mental and physical health. Our interests can also give us a sense of purpose, especially when they align with our personal values. Someone who cares about the environment, for instance, might get into organic gardening, upcycling, or volunteering, all of which influence their identity as an environmentally conscious person. Our hobbies and interests, then, are a crucial part of what defines us as people.

You might, however, question where disability comes into this discussion of hobbies. If you acquire a disability, or if your disability has become more severe, the challenge comes when it makes it difficult for you to participate in interests which were previously important to you. So, what can we do if this happens? It can be a really crushing blow if you can no longer pursue something you used to enjoy, and which was important to your identity. As we discussed in the first chapter, when your life undergoes a major change and you can no longer do the things you loved, it is natural to feel angry and even to grieve your life before disability. The same applies here. If there was something that you loved and that made you feel alive every time that you did it, then I am sorry that you can no longer do the thing which made your heart sing. Such grief is a perfectly natural process, and if you're looking for tips to help with this, the first chapter is a great start.

So, your disability might interfere with how you can practice your hobbies and interests. What is the solution? Just because you have a disability, it does not mean that the world of hobbies is entirely inaccessible to you. Trust me, I know – I really do – that you might feel there is nothing in life that can replace the thing that you were so passionate about. I used to be an avid drummer, something which became increasingly impossible as my joints weakened, and my neurological issues worsened. At the time, it felt like my friends and family couldn't understand how huge this blow felt, and I spiralled into a pit of depression where I was convinced that I would never find anything that I would be so passionate about again. But as time passed and my depression eased, I became more open to the world and was willing to try different hobbies that were more accessible for me. There are now so many things that I am passionate about, from writing, to volunteering, to crocheting, to crafting, and swimming. In time, you will discover that there are many ways to adapt your favourites pastimes around your disability, even though sometimes you might have to think a little creatively about how to do it. Alternatively, there are many adaptive and disability-friendly hobbies to get involved in, so you could even try different interests to discover a new passion!

Making space for the things you enjoy

Returning to or acquiring a hobby might seem easier said than done, especially if you have a disability that limits your energy or raises your pain and fatigue levels. Even people with the same diagnosis can have vastly different energy reserves or levels of pain, depending on the severity of their condition. For some, incorporating a hobby into their day might feel like a bit of a struggle, whilst for others it might seem completely impossible if you need to use the little energy that you have just to survive from day to day.

If you're in this situation with your disability or chronic illness, you might have concerned family members and friends suggesting anything they can think of to improve your daily life. Much to your frustration, the very thing they may suggest is to look for a new hobby that can distract you from your pain and fatigue. I'd be willing to bet a fair amount that someone has either suggested that you try yoga or audiobooks by now. Your loved ones' advice might initially seem hurtful to you; they seemingly do not understand the depths of your pain and fatigue which are making it impossible to just survive, let alone thrive and pursue a new hobby. Again, I know how upsetting, frustrating, and isolating it can be when those who you love just don't seem to comprehend your life with a disability. Trust me too, though, that their advice comes from a good and empathetic place. It is hard for those who love you to see you struggle, and they will just be concerned with helping you to have the best quality of life possible, in whatever form that now looks like for you. The sources of your joy might now differ to your life pre-disability, but it is still possible to make space and find enjoyment as a disabled person.

This fact can be a very difficult one to acknowledge and accept, especially when things are at their hardest at the start of your journey with disability. However, as you learn to manage your condition better with the help of pacing and other management tools (see chapter eight for further details), you will hopefully feel a little less overwhelmed. You may find that, each day, it becomes a little bit easier to carry your pain and fatigue. Making space and pacing your energy for the things that bring you joy can make life as a disabled person so much more bearable.

The core aim of this chapter is to encourage you to re-engage with your interests and passions in a way that is safe, sustainable, and manageable for you given your different circumstances. The remainder of this chapter will consider different hobbies and interests, and how these are accessible or can be adapted to different access needs. We will also think about how to fit joy into your life if you have an energy-limiting condition and consider which hobbies might be suitable or could be adapted to be low-energy. You can still incorporate your passions into your life with a disability and, if not, there's a whole new host of accessible and low-energy hobbies that are just waiting for you to discover!

Sports and physical activity

Nowadays, there is a great variety of sports and physical activities which are accessible, or which can be adapted for people with a variety of disabilities. There are several different types of adaptive wheelchairs and equipment which have been specifically designed to make sport accessible. Sports clubs can often provide this specialist equipment on loan, or they may be able to help with grants towards buying your own equipment, especially if you reach a competitive level. When I started wheelchair rugby with a local club, I fell in love instantly and knew I wanted to be part of the team one day. I soon began paying subs and my club assigned me a rugby wheelchair which would remain mine for as long as I stayed with the club. Wheelchair rugby was a great sport for me; it got me moving in a way that was accessible, I enjoyed the exercise, and it was so nice to interact with other disabled people and wheelchair users who just got what I was going through. Some other accessible sports include:

- **Wheelchair basketball.** Wheelchair basketball has been a Paralympic sport since 1960. It is like regular basketball, except that players are strapped into specially designed wheelchairs which allow for agility, precision, and sharp turns. It is played on a full regulation court, and the basket is at the same height as for regular basketball. As a team sport, it can grow leadership and teamworking skills, as well as developing social relationships and strategic thinking.

- **Football.** Football can be adapted for different disabilities. Blind football has teams of five and is really an adapted version of futsal. Outfield players must be registered as blind, although goal keepers can be either fully or partially sighted. To ensure a fair playing field, all outfield players must wear eye patches or shades if they have a level of light or shape perception. The ball is adapted with metal shards sewn inside, which create noise when the ball is moving so players can locate it. The aim is the same as regular football – to score as many goals in the opposing team's net as possible. Football can further be adapted for those who are amputees or who have a limb difference. Players use a pair of crutches to move about the pitch and – at grassroots level – you can choose whether to use your prosthesis as well, if you have one. Walking football has become popular with amputee players too, and helps players of all ages who want a less intense form of the game to participate.

- **Wheelchair rugby.** Wheelchair rugby (WC rugby) became a Paralympic sport in 2000. It is a team sport for disabled players and is one of the few sports where all genders can play on the same team. Specially adapted sports wheelchairs are used as WC rugby is a full-contact sport, meaning that players can make contact with each other's wheelchairs but not their bodies. The goal is to carry the ball across the other team's try line, like regular rugby. WC rugby is sometimes called by its nickname 'Murderball', due to its aggressive play and the propensity for noisy contact, punctured tires, and flipped wheelchairs. There is a different variant called wheelchair rugby league (WCL), which is an adapted version of rugby league football, and which has its own distinct set of rules. WCL is more inclusive, as it allows disabled and non-disabled players to participate together on the same team.

- **Adaptive cycling.** There are many different types of adaptive cycles available for a range of disabilities and access needs. Recumbent cycles and trikes can help you to pedal when seated in a slightly laid-back position with your legs stretched out in front. Hand cycles allow you to use your hands to pedal and are a great option for people who either cannot use their legs at all or who have limited power and strength in their lower limbs. You can also get hand-trike attachments which clamp onto your own wheelchair, saving on storage space and supporting you to go out independently whenever you need; these kinds of attachment work best on active-style wheelchairs. Trikes have three wheels and are a lot sturdier than traditional bikes, so can aid those who have balance problems. If you need the support of a carer or a cycling companion to help keep you safe, a tandem bike might be the one for you. Or, if you need a little help to get around tricky terrain, power-assisted bikes could be the choice for you, as they can give you a little extra boost of power when you need it. Adaptive cycles can be pricey, so it is often worth checking with Cycling UK to see if they have any local schemes where you can try different cycles out, so that you can participate in recreational or competitive cycling.

- **Adaptive dance.** Dance is a great hobby for many disabled people, and it can be easily adapted to suit someone's access requirements. It can lead to improvements for your heart, your bones and joints, your range of motion, your stamina and your emotional expression. Dances can be adapted using mobility aids - such as crutches, wheelchairs, or prostheses - or for people with sensory and learning disabilities. If you're interested in adaptive dance, it might be worth checking out Kate Stanforth (@katestanforth) and the Kate Stanforth dance academy (@katestanforthdance), an online studio run by disabled dancer and model Kate; sessions are led by other disabled dance teachers who have adapted their choreography for a whole host of disabilities. You could alternatively look for Chelsie Hill (@chelsiehill), Kaylee Bays (@slayleebays) and the Rollettes

(@rollettes_la), who are disabled choreographers, and part of the Rollettes disabled dance team based in Los Angeles. Dance for disabled people has grown in popularity in recent years, not least with disabled contestants such as actress Rose Ayling-Ellis and comedian Chris McCausland winning popular dance competition and entertainment programme *Strictly Come Dancing* on the BBC.

- **Wheelchair tennis.** Wheelchair tennis has been played at all four Grand Slams – the Australian Open, Wimbledon, Roland Garros and the American Open - since 2007 and became a Paralympic sport in 1988. Players use specifically adapted manual wheelchairs to manoeuvre about the court and are divided into two classes. The Open class comprises players with a physical disability affecting one or both legs, but who have retained their arm function. The Quad class is for players with a disability affecting their playing arm. Many of the rules are the same as for regular tennis, except that the wheelchair user can allow the ball to bounce twice before having to hit it with their racket. You do not have to be a full-time wheelchair user to play or compete either; many players are ambulatory wheelchair users, meaning that they can stand and walk in some capacity but need a wheelchair for the remainder of the time. If a player cannot handle a manual wheelchair with their disability, they may be offered a powered one.

- **Gym and weightlifting.** For those who enjoy spending time in the gym, you can still do this with a disability – you may just need a few adaptations. Gyms can provide equipment that can be adjusted to help people with various disabilities, such as straps to help with holding weights or wheelchair-accessible gym machines like hand-bikes. There is a lot of gym equipment which may already be accessible, including resistance bands, kettlebells, and gym balls. In the first instance, it might help to get yourself a personal trainer and speak to them about your disabilities and any physical adaptations you might now need. Your trainer can then produce a workout regime for you that will help you to reach your fitness goals. You could equally speak to gym instructors to see if they can make any of the gym classes accessible to you. If you love to work out, but the gym isn't really your scene, there are plenty of home workouts online that you can adapt to your needs. The Wheel with Me Adapt Fit app has several accessible workout routines and Adapt to Perform on YouTube creates adapted workout routines with basic gym equipment or everyday household objects.

- **Sitting volleyball.** Sitting volleyball first appeared at the Paralympic games in 1976 and is very inclusive. It is a competitive team sport at club level, played with mixed-gender teams of disabled and non-disabled athletes sitting on the floor. The game is far from stationery, though! Whilst athletes must maintain contact between their pelvis and the floor, the game is fast paced, requires agility, and utilises the same skills and techniques as standing volleyball. Sitting volleyball affords you plenty of opportunities to work on your overall fitness and, as a team sport, you can get to know new people as well. You could play the sport for its social and recreational benefits, or you can play at a more competitive level if you wish. Sitting volleyball can be a rewarding and enjoyable sport, and there are plenty of clubs across the UK which are open to new players.

- **Para Ice Hockey.** Para ice hockey is sometimes known as sledge hockey and has been a winter Paralympic sport since 1994. It was created for people with disabilities affecting their lower limbs and is played on sledges with a pair of special spiked sticks which allow players navigate across the ice. It is an exciting and physically demanding sport, which is perhaps why it has become one of the most-watched sports of the Winter Paralympics. At club level in the UK, para ice hockey is open to players aged 18 and over, with disabled and non-disabled people playing alongside one another. Teams can be found in Cambridge, Cardiff, Manchester, and Sheffield to name a few, and clubs typically have some spare equipment for those who wish to come along to sessions to try the sport out.

- **Swimming.** Swimming is an accessible sport for people with a range of disabilities, and can improve balance, strength, mental health, and overall fitness. At competitive level, it has been a Paralympic sport since the 1960s. Moving your body in water can be incredibly therapeutic and give greater freedom to those with limited mobility. Many pools are now equipped with hoists to help disabled people to get in and out of the pool, and some have submersible wheelchairs so you can enter the pool safely. Swimming is a great source of physiotherapy for those with conditions that affect their joints, especially if you can get some specialist hydrotherapy support. Some councils in the UK run schemes that offer one-to-one or group lessons for adults with additional needs or learning disabilities and might offer free swimming for you and your carer if you receive the higher components of Personal Independence Payment (PIP) for your disability.

- **Wheelchair fencing.** Wheelchair fencing was one of the original Paralympic sports in the 1960s and is a dynamic sport to either watch or participate in. Two fencers compete against one another in wheelchairs that are fixed in position on the piste, and they must keep at least one half of their buttocks on the wheelchair seat. Athletes with certain disabilities can participate at a competitive level, including those with spinal cord injuries, lower-leg amputees, those with cerebral palsy, and others with physical disabilities that require a wheelchair. Like its standing counterpart, wheelchair fencing requires technique, style, and precision and is a great sport to practice if you'd like to improve your agility and reflexes. There are three modified weapons from which you can choose, which are the foil, epee and sabre. They are used to score points on specific areas of the body, depending on the chosen weapon.

- **Adapted hockey.** Adapted hockey is a mixed-gender team sport which can be played by athletes with varying degrees of disability. It can either be played in a manual or an electric

69

wheelchair and athletes use one of two types of sticks: the conventional hockey stick or the t-stick, which features plastic blades located at the front of the chair. As a team sport, adapted hockey is great for social interaction, getting to know new like-minded people, and improving your mental wellbeing. The aim of the game is the same as regular hockey, which is to score as many goals against the opposing team as possible. Adapted hockey therefore fosters skills such as strategic thinking, leadership, and the ability to work together as a team to succeed.

- **Disability sailing.** Sailing is a fun and social outdoor activity that lets you be at the heart of nature, both battling the elements and learning to work with the rhythms of the natural world. Sailing is inclusive of an array of disabilities, as there is a wide range of boats and sailing equipment that can support disabled people to get out onto the water and achieve independence. For example, sailing boats can be specially adapted with joysticks and other equipment to allow disabled people to operate them independently. As well as traditional sailing, you could try rowing, canoeing, kayaking, windsurfing, or canal boating until you find something which ignites your passion! There are several local clubs across the UK which offer facilities for disabled sailors, so you could find one near to you. The Royal Yachting Association also runs the Sailability Programme, which supports disabled people to get into sailing and increases opportunities for disabled sailors to race and train both locally and nationally.

- **Boccia.** Boccia became a Paralympic sport in 1984 and is related to bowls and pétanque. Players can compete as individuals, pairs, or teams of three in mixed-gender events. It is a precision ball sport, where players aim to throw soft leather balls as close as they can to a white ball, or jack. Boccia is inclusive for players with diverse disabilities, as the ball can be moved with hands, feet, or with the help of an assistive ramp or head pointer. Points are accumulated depending on which team's balls are closest to the jack, and the team with the most points at the end will be the winners. Boccia tests muscle control and accuracy but requires strategic thinking and incredible skill too. The tactics of the sport create great tension and excitement! To find out how to get involved, Boccia England is a registered charity and their website has a wealth of information, including a search tool to help you to find a club local to you.

- **Para-climbing.** Para-climbing has been confirmed as a Paralympic sport for 2028. To have as fair a competition as possible, athletes are put into different categories depending on their disability and how much it affects their ability to undertake the necessary activities involved in para-climbing. So, for example, blind climbers cannot compete against climbers in wheelchairs. People with certain disabilities can receive different support whilst climbing; for instance, partially sighted climbers can have a sighted guide instructing them from the ground, whilst leg amputees can choose whether to wear a prosthesis. In competitions, climbers' rankings are based on the furthest height they reach and those with the highest scores will win.

- **Track and field events.** Disabled athletes can take part in track and field events with various adaptations to support them. For field events including javelin, discus, and shotput, athletes are often seated on throwing frames which allow them to use the same throwing equipment as non-disabled athletes. Track events include wheelchair racing, in which athletes use specially designed wheelchairs which can race on the road or on a track. Wheelchair racing is open to any athletes with a qualifying disability such as amputees, spinal cord injuries, cerebral palsy, and so forth. Athletes are classified according to the nature and severity of their disability. The British Wheelchair Racing Association (BWRA) is the governing body for wheelchair racing and adaptive field athletics in the UK. Their website has a tool to find a club local to you.

- **Adaptive archery.** Adaptive archery is a an accessible, inclusive, and social sport. Most disabilities can be accommodated and, whatever your age or ability, you can shoot in a social setting, where disabled and non-disabled archers join together. You can even enter intra- and inter-club competitions. Disabled archers can either shoot standing, or on a perch stool or sitting down. Archery GB is the British body for archery and has over 800 clubs, which either shoot outdoors, indoors, or a mixture of both depending on the seasons. If you'd like to give archery a try, clubs often hold 'Have a Go' taster sessions, or you could book onto a beginner's course.

These courses teach you all the basics of how to shoot, score, and assemble equipment safely.

- **Goalball.** Goalball became a Paralympic sport in 1976 and was developed following the Second World War to help rehabilitate disabled veterans who were blind or partially sighted. Today, sighted athletes can compete if they are blindfolded whilst playing. In fact, to ensure that the game is fair, all players must wear opaque eye shades. Goalball is played by teams of six, with three players on the court at any one time. The aim is to get the ball past your opponents and into their net to score. The ball is only ever thrown, not kicked, and players remain on their hands and knees whilst playing and defending their net. It is a fast-paced and action-packed sport that is fun either for its players or those spectating and commentating.

- **Bowls.** Bowls is one of the most inclusive sports for players with or without disabilities. Recently, the game has become far more accessible for those with disabilities with the introduction of different wheelchairs and accessible equipment. A full list of adaptive equipment can be found on the Disability Bowls England website. Bowls can be played in many configurations, including singles, pairs, triples or fours, so offers great opportunities to socialise with other players. If you want to get competitive, you can play at club, county, or even national level to represent the UK at the Commonwealth Games. Disability Bowls England is the national charity working to promote bowls and encourage more disabled people to try this sport. They hold taster sessions at clubs throughout

73

the year, so it's worth keeping an eye on their website for the latest updates.

- **Equestrian.** The Riding for the Disabled Association (RDA) is a great place to start if you're looking to get involved in equestrian sports as a disabled person. RDA offers a wide range of activities for those of all ages and abilities, including riding, carriage driving, showjumping, vaulting, dressage, and endurance. Equestrian sports are sometimes recommended by medical professionals for physiotherapy; the specific branch is called hippotherapy, where the movement of the horse is used to improve a person's mental and physical health, as well as their balance and posture. If you wish to take the sport to a competitive level, RDA runs regional and national competitions, as well as riding holidays and educational programmes. These are great ways to socialise with other riders, make new friends, and have fun with your horse.

- **Other sports you may be interested in:** badminton, cricket, cue sports, curling, fishing, golf, gymnastics, martial arts, para-triathlon, pickle ball, shooting, snow sports, table tennis, water skiing, and yoga.

Sports are great, but they aren't for everyone

Sports and exercise are important for maintaining our mental wellbeing, social interaction, and overall physical health; working on these things can be even more important as we learn to adapt to being disabled, especially to stay healthy and connect with other people who share similar interests and experiences. Sport isn't for everyone, though, and that's perfectly ok. I wasn't an overly sporty kid and enjoyed crafty hobbies much more. When my disability first became more severe, though, I was hugely fatigued and in so much pain that I could barely manage to get out of bed, let alone go for a run or play a round of tennis. Even as my energy started to come back a little bit, I still had to pace carefully and not over-exert myself, meaning that I had to look for other, lower-energy hobbies to occupy my time.

For those with energy-limiting conditions, such as ME/ CFS and Long COVID, sport might even be inadvisable. It can be difficult to exercise when you must deal with the consequences of post-exertional malaise (PEM) and spend days resting to recover. The remainder of this chapter will look at other, lower-energy hobbies and how to adapt them around various disabilities, to give you some other ideas of where you can find moments of joy:

- **Knitting and crochet.** Knitting uses two needles and crochet uses a hook, but both take a ball of yarn to create textiles. There are plenty of starter kits and videos available on the internet to get you started, but you could instead look for classes at your local craft shop or community centre. For those with joint issues, you can easily buy ergonomic needles and hooks. If you have limited dexterity, there are videos online that can teach you how to crochet one-handed or ReMAP – a UK charity which provides custom-made adaptive equipment to disabled people free of charge – has devised a one-handed knitting aid. You could instead explore a Kroh's crochet aid, created for people with MS, arthritis, or other neurological conditions, to help you to keep the tension in your yarn. Knitting and crochet are easy hobbies to pace for those with energy-limiting conditions, as they can be easily picked up and put down depending on how you're feeling.

- **Sewing.** Sewing is another great hobby for people with energy-limiting conditions. Projects are easy to pick-up and put down if you get fatigued, and you could even work on multiple projects at once, so at any one time you can choose the project that best fits how much energy you have left on that day. Alternatively, you could batch tasks to prevent you hopping from one to another, so you could do all your pinning work in one go, then your cutting work, then your sewing and so on. To manage your energy, you could sew in short 30-minute bursts with rest breaks in between to better pace yourself. With regards to adaptive equipment, try to find what works best for you as, depending on your disability and your needs, some hacks may work better for you than others. If you struggle with hand dexterity, you can get Prym easy grip pins that are easier to grasp than traditional pins. You could invest in some Fiskars easy-grip snips or spring-loaded scissors to make cutting fabric and threads easier. If you struggle with pressing, you could try a silicone mat underneath the fabric to make the motion of ironing smoother and to reduce the strain on the arm and elbow. If ironing itself is difficult, you will likely be better suited to a steamer than a conventional iron. If you find threading a needle tricky, you might try a Clover desktop needle threader to help you out. There are many more hacks that you can find out about from other sewers online.

- **Cross-stitch or embroidery.** Embroidery uses a needle to stitch yarn or thread to decorate fabrics, and cross-stitch is a form of counted-thread embroidery with x-shaped stitches. Cross-stitch and embroidery are good hobbies for those with little energy, as they can be easily picked up and put down depending on your fatigue levels. There are several adaptations you can implement to make these crafts more accessible. You could use larger needles or a coarser, lower-count Aida fabric on which to stitch your designs. In addition, you could use thicker embroidery floss for better grip and visibility. There is also specialised equipment available, including needle threaders and hoop holders. Good lighting and magnification might help if you are partially sighted, and you could find large print or colour coded patterns to make them easier to read. If you want to get started with cross-stitch or embroidery, there are plenty of kits which can teach you the basic stitches and where everything comes pre-measured, which is great for reducing the amount of energy required. You could investigate classes at your local craft store too, which could be a great way to meet new and like-minded people.

- **Pottery.** Pottery uses clay to make objects such as bowls, containers, or decorative objects, which are then hardened by air-drying or by using heat. It is one of the oldest and most widespread of the decorative arts. Pottery can be an incredibly relaxing and expressive hobby. It is also a good choice for those with disabilities and chronic illness, as it allows you to be creative whilst conserving your energy. There are various adaptations you can use to make it even more accessible for you. You could start with Fimo or air-drying clay and use techniques such as coil-building which do not require a wheel. There are plenty of starter kits for this, such as Sculpd or Pott'd, which include all the tools you'll need and pre-measured clay; this can save energy and means you can easily get it out and tidy it away. If you do want to get into throwing, you can get adaptive wheels that allow you to sit rather than stand, as well as hand levers instead of foot pedals to help you control the speed of the wheel. If you want a low-energy version of throwing, you could get into miniature pottery. Small Ceramics offers tiny pottery wheels to enable you to make small creations which can be fired in the microwave, and which can be a great energy-saving alternative to traditional throwing. If you want to get started, starter kits are a great way to go. Alternatively, you could check out online tutorials or local classes, especially if you want to get to know others in your community.

- **Origami.** Origami is a Japanese art of paper folding. It can be enjoyed by people with diverse disabilities, such as blind or partially sighted people, as there are plenty of tutorials online which are accessible for screen readers. Origami is easy to pick up and tidy away, and you can do it all from the comfort of your own home, so

78

is great for those with energy-limiting conditions. There are plenty of books, starter kits and an abundance of tutorials online or in-person if you want to start, or you could look at classes at your local craft shop. You could even pick-up pre-cut origami sheets of paper in an array of colours and designs, to further save time and precious energy.

- **Painting, drawing, and photography.** Painting, drawing, and photography are fantastic hobbies for those with disabilities, as they allow you to express yourself and how you are feeling in a safe and controlled manner. There is a lot that you can do to make painting more accessible for your needs. You could give adaptive weighted or lightweight brushes a try to help with greater control or hand tremors or use specialised grips for those with poor dexterity. For watercolour painting, there are refillable paint brushes and no-spill contained ones to prevent spills. Adjustable easels can accommodate different heights and angles to suit your sitting position. You could also create digital art by zooming in and out on sections on an iPAD or tablet or making sure your images are well back-lit, techniques which can help to create art for partially sighted artists. If you're looking for some inspiration, or if your love of art solely extends to admiring it, there are so many disabled artists out there, including: Paul Castle, Clara Woods, Alison Lapper, David Hockney, Angela de la Cruz, or Yayoi Kusama.

- **Videography.** Videography is the art of making video films. Given recent advances in technology, videography can now easily be achieved with our everyday gadgets. You can still get specialist equipment if you need, or you could just use your mobile phone with its accessibility adaptations such as screen-readers. There are plenty of tutorials and blogs online and on social media, which offer tips on how to make better videos or how to edit. You could investigate at your local community centre or college for classes too. There is free editing software available on the app store. This means that you can edit anytime and anywhere that's comfortable for you, which is convenient to manage your energy reserves. Remember, your videos do not have to be long or even qualify as short films; social media has recently opened up the possibility of posting shorter 'reel' films, which can be equally – or if not more – impactful as longer films.

- **Baking and cooking.** Baking and cooking can be quite a meditative and creative way to relax. Whilst it can take a bit more time and energy than other hobbies, there are various adjustments you can implement to make it more accessible to you. You could use adaptive equipment such as electronic can openers, weighted or light-weight utensils, automatic vegetable choppers, or switch-activated scissors for those whose disability affects their hands, or talking scales and liquid measures for those who are blind or partially sighted. You could make adaptations to your kitchen, such as lowering countertops so that wheelchairs can get under or install perch or swivel stools to help you to save energy. For those with energy limiting conditions, you could group and pace different tasks with rests in between, such as doing all your measuring, then chopping, then mixing and so forth. Whilst it can be nice to bake everything from scratch, pre-made packet mixes can help to save time and reduce fatigue on low-energy days. It can also be helpful to batch cook on your better days and freeze portions or doughs that you can easily defrost and bake on worse days to save your energy and reduce symptoms.

- **Journaling or scrapbooking.** Journalling is about writing down your thoughts, feelings, and experiences, whilst scrapbooking involves organising photos and memories into a book and embellishing them. It can be a very relaxing, creative, and meditative hobby, and you could check out your local craft shop or community centre for classes to get you started. There is a swathe of adaptive equipment you can find to help you. Pencil grips, jumbo pens or crayons, and the FUNctionalhand tool can all support you to get better grip. There are textured paint brushes, easy-grip scissors, stencils, or stickers to assist you too. If you're blind or partially sighted, you can still get involved in the fun of journaling or scrapbooking. You could make an audio journal using a voice recorder on your phone or use a Braille writer and sticky back paper to create messages to include in a scrapbook. You might want to use more tactile elements such as textured card, corrugated paper, different fabrics, buttons and gems, or you may even wish to include different scents that you associate with particular memories in your scrapbook using perfumes and essential oils.

- **Reading.** Many people find enjoyment in reading and with the growth of technology in recent years, there are now many more ways to read than before. If you find it difficult to hold conventional, heavy books, you could consider a book cushion or using an e-reader and stand to hold your books for you. E-readers can be a great option for people with disabilities; they are easy to hold, you can increase the text size for people who are partially sighted or who get brain fog and eye strain, and you can get different versions to be back-lit or not depending on your preference. And they allow you to carry as many books as you want at once! If you are blind or partially sighted, the Royal National Institute of the Blind (RNIB) have many audiobooks, large print, and Braille books available. Audiobooks have grown in popularity over the past few years with the introduction of platforms such as Audible (Amazon), Spotify, and Libby. For those with energy limiting conditions, it can help to pace your reading, such as resting between chapters or different sections of the book.

- **Podcasts.** A podcast is an episodic series of audio-programmes which you can listen to or download from the internet. Today, there are so many different podcasts in numerous languages which cover diverse topics, from comedy, to mindful living, to true crime and beyond. Whatever grabs your interest, you're bound to find a podcast that you like. Podcasts are accessible for disabled people, especially for the blind or partially sighted and for people with energy-limiting conditions; you can easily turn them on or off again as needed to rest, or you could pace yourself between different episodes. You can listen to podcasts whilst you're doing other tasks, such as the dishes, walking to the shops, or putting the washing machine on, so they can help to distract your mind from tasks which are fatiguing or painful. Some of the most popular podcast platforms include Spotify, Apple Pod, BBC Sounds, and Podbean.

-   **Sporting fanbases and commentating sports.** Whilst physically doing sports might not be suitable for everyone, this doesn't mean that you must leave the sporting world behind you altogether. Those who were once avid athletes can still find enjoyment and fulfilment as part of the sport's fanbase. If you have a favourite sportsperson, team, or sport, you could follow them by watching events on television – especially good for low energy days – or attending live events if you feel up to it. You could combine this with other hobbies and create a scrapbook about your sport, volunteer to support the team in other ways, write blogs about the sport, or even learn to commentate, or create your own podcast about it. If you feel up to it, you might even wish to attend gatherings with other fans with whom you can socialise and connect. Indeed, no longer being able to participate yourself might be the gateway to engaging with a sport in an alternative, yet equally fulfilling, manner.

-   **Visiting museums and art galleries.** In a similar vein, if you do not always feel like you have the energy to create art for yourself, you could still engage with this hobby by visiting art galleries. Or, if there is a particular topic that you are passionate about – such as World War history – you could visit museums to find out more about your special interest. If you are struggling with pain or fatigue, many museums and galleries have places that you can sit dotted around the exhibits, or they have mobility aids and wheelchairs that you can borrow whilst you're there, helping to make your experience more accessible. You could again combine your museum or gallery visits with other hobbies, and create scrapbooks, podcasts, or blogs about your interests and experiences. For particularly low energy days, since the COVID-19 pandemic, quite a few museums and galleries have created virtual tours that you can enjoy from the comfort of your own home, and which you could pace throughout the day according to your needs.

- **Gardening.** There are so many benefits to gardening, including spending time in nature, boosting your mental health, or relieving feelings of stress or anxiety. As we age, gardening has been shown to be beneficial for protecting your memory, supporting your immune system's functionality, and fostering feelings of connection if you garden with others.[9] Although gardening might not initially seem like a very accessible hobby due to its physicality, there are several things that you can do to make it more suited to your needs. For those with joint pain, there are ergonomic tools to reduce the

---

[9] Healthline. (20 June 2025) 9 Benefits of Gardening, plus helpful tips [Online]. Available at https://www.healthline.com/health/healthful-benefits-of-gardening (Accessed 8 August 2025).

strain on your hands or wrists, or you could use a garden kneeler, which is a foam pad that protects the knees during prolonged periods. You could alternatively raise garden beds or use raised trugs to make planting, digging, and weeding easier, or employ long-reach tools to allow you to tend your plants from a standing or seated position, such as in a wheelchair. To transport items, you could use mobility aids such as rollators or purchase a collapsible garden bucket, which is easier to transport on a wheelchair than a conventional, cumbersome bucket. If you need easy access to water, you could install a water table or a water-collecting reservoir. As you design your garden, plan to create safe, stable paths with a non-slip surface and which are wide enough to accommodate wheelchairs or other mobility equipment. Finally, if you are blind or partially sighted, you could position lights at key points, use tactile paving, or place landmark items to help you to navigate around the garden.

- **Listening to or playing music.** Playing or listening to music can have many benefits, as well as making us feel relaxed and bringing us enjoyment. It can improve your memory and increase your self-confidence, in addition to improving your mood and reducing stress and anxiety. Listening to music is typically not too taxing for those with energy-limiting conditions, provided that it isn't too loud as this might trigger noise sensitivities. Depending on your disability, though, it might feel like it is impossible to be involved in playing music, for instance, if you are d/Deaf or hard of hearing. But, thanks to recent innovations, there are things that you can try so that making music is more accessible to you. If you struggle to hold an instrument, you could use microphone stands, Velcro or self-adherent bandages to keep your instrument in place. You could instead adapt the instrument itself, such as glueing popsicle sticks to piano keys to extend them or using pipe insulation to make drum sticks easier to grasp. The One-Handed Musical Instrument Trust (OHMI) adapts instruments for physically disabled musicians with only one upper limb. Such small adaptations can have a huge impact on your ability to play the instrument. You could instead change the technique needed to play an instrument if it is easier for your needs, such as using the right hand to play at the top of the recorder rather than the left if this works better for you and your disability. In addition to these hacks, there have recently been plenty of innovative inventions to encourage more disabled musicians. The MiMu gloves – developed by musician Imogen Heap – are wearable gesture-controlled gloves which allow musicians with disabilities to compose and perform music by making certain gestures. The Skoog is a box-shaped accessible instrument which you press or squeeze using different parts of your body to create sounds. It is fully customisable via the Skoog app, so you can make different sounds depending on how the instrument is manipulated. It can therefore improve motor skills and co-ordination, whilst allowing the musician to explore their musical expression. The EyeHarp is a musical instrument which can be played with movements of the eyes or neck. It utilises eye-tracking software and computer software to create a pentatonic or heptatonic scale, from which the musician can then play and compose. It gives paralysed musicians and those who cannot use or control their limbs the opportunity to play in ensembles with others. The Soundbeam is an interactive MIDI device which detects movement of the hands with ultrasonic beams and turns it into sounds from which musicians can create melodies. It has been incredibly useful for people with cerebral palsy, Down's syndrome, and other learning disabilities. Finally, for those who are d/Deaf or hard of hearing, Subpac is a great piece of equipment to include them in the experience of enjoying music. It is a wearable device which looks like a vest, and it creates an immersive musical experience by transferring deep bass frequencies onto the body, thereby transforming a piece of music into a full corporeal experience.

- **Jigsaws, puzzles and Lego.** Jigsaws, puzzles, boardgames, and Lego can be fun and accessible for a range of disabilities. For those with-energy-limiting conditions, jigsaws and puzzles can be easy to pace and to put away and get out, especially with the help of rollable puzzle mats. The Royal National Institute for the Blind (RNIB) has many adapted jigsaws, puzzles, and boardgames for those who are blind or partially sighted. This includes Braille playing cards, tactile dominoes, Braille Scrabble, and many others. Catherine Daley has designed puzzles with key-shaped pieces, which make it possible to do the puzzle by feel alone, although it also includes bright colouring and yellow edges for those who are partially sighted to see. Puzzles for Everybody™ are designed to be tactile and sensory and so are playable by people with varying disabilities. In 2020, Lego launched Braille bricks to support blind and partially sighted players to build and exercise their imagination.

- **Videogaming.** Since the launch of gaming consoles in the 1970s, videogaming has become an increasingly popular hobby and is now a multi-billion-dollar industry. With this growing market, developers have recently begun to cater to disabled gamers and to make gaming more accessible for them. Here are some tips to help you make sure the games you're choosing are as accessible as possible and that you're making the most out of the experience as a disabled gamer. You could check that text is easy to read using large font and higher contrast, and that sound feedback and audio narration are provided, especially for those who are partially sighted. You could check that subtitles and closed captions are included, especially for any key dialogue between characters. Content warnings should be given via audio and text throughout the game where appropriate. In terms of gaming hardware, Xbox is one of the top videogaming companies for accessibility. Xbox have a set of best practice guidelines for accessibility and for improving the experience for disabled gamers, which are publicly available. Their adaptive controller and hub can be customised to each player's needs. This allows gamers with limited mobility to have an alternative means of interacting with the game, and it can even connect to outside devices like wheelchair joysticks. The Xbox adaptive controller was designed by gamer Spencer Allen, who became paralysed after an accident. PlayStation have an adaptive controller too, which was developed for disabled people with limited dexterity. For those with energy-limiting conditions, you could switch to lighter hand-held consoles such as the Nintendo Switch or the Steam Deck and pace yourself between matches or levels. If you're looking for accessible games, CanIPlayThat.com reviews video games for accessibility and hosts the Annual Accessibility Awards. Gaming is a fantastic hobby that can help you to meet and socialise with others from the comfort of your own home through online and collaborative playing options. Videogaming can improve dexterity and accuracy, response times, strategy and leadership, and communication skills, and can encourage teamwork and critical thinking, as well as boosting your mood and reducing stress.

- **Volunteering.** Volunteering allows you to make a positive difference in the world and help others, as well as giving you opportunities to improve your self-esteem, confidence, and well-being. If there is a particular cause that you are passionate about – such as the environment, education, or supporting others with disabilities – there are so many charities and organisations out there who will be looking for volunteers for all kinds of roles. Volunteering can be a great way to build up your skills and confidence, especially if you're looking to go back into the workplace. But even if you are just hoping to get involved with a great cause, volunteering can be a fantastic option for those with energy-limiting conditions as many roles now are flexible and you can choose to do as much or as little as you like. Since the COVID-19 pandemic, certain volunteering roles have adapted to the hybrid world and so you might find that there are plenty of roles you can do from the comfort of your own home and pace as you need. Whether online or in person, volunteering is a great way to meet other like-minded people and build social connections. If you would like to get started with volunteering, try writing down things you are passionate about and search for charities local to you or online which fit that profile. Sometimes you may need to apply for a volunteering role, so having an up-to-date CV which details your skills can be handy.

- **Learning a language.** Learning a different language or learning British sign language (BSL) is a great way to connect with other people and communities online and around the world. As a hobby, it is easy to adapt to your access needs. There are plenty of free apps that you can download onto a tablet or phone to help you learn a new language from wherever you wish, such as Duolingo, Babbel, or Rosetta Stone. Their learning modules are often broken down into shorter lessons, so you can choose just how much you feel able to do in one sitting and at a time of the day that works best for you. If you would like to enhance your language learning, you could look for local lessons or opportunities to practice speaking that language with other learners or native speakers, which is a great way to improve your skills and grow your confidence. If that option isn't available or accessible to you, you could instead listen to TV, radio, podcasts, and audiobooks in your chosen language to really immerse yourself in another culture and turn off the subtitles as your understanding improves. Learning a language is a fantastic way to build relationships with others, so you could search online for a pen friend from another country and, eventually, maybe even visit them!

- **Bird watching.** Bird watching – sometimes called 'twitching' – is an incredibly calming pastime, which can stimulate your senses and support your mental health. It can strengthen your connection to nature, which has many benefits in terms of lowering stress and anxiety. Bird watching is a fabulous way to pass the time for those with disabilities. You can take part in local accessible parks or wildlife reserves, or even from the comfort of your home. You could set up a bird feeder or plant bird-friendly flora in your garden or on your balcony to encourage the birds to visit, then sit back and relax as you watch them fluttering past. Bird watching does not require great energy reserves and can be paced with rest breaks in between for those with energy-limiting conditions. If you would like to socialise with others, there are plenty of bird-watching blogs and message threads online, or you could search for a club in your local area where you can meet other 'twitchers'. If you would like to get started, there are many books, websites, and apps – such as Merling – that can help you with identifying birds from their appearance or song. You could also combine 'twitching' with other hobbies and create a journal or scrapbook with all your sightings of the different breeds of bird you have seen or would like to see.

- **Other hobbies you might like to try.** Model making, quilting, calligraphy, graphic design, woodworking, dog training for obedience or agility, raising pets, pool and snooker, creative writing, poetry, blogging, collecting, astronomy, stargazing, geocaching, fantasy sports leagues, reenactment… the world is your oyster!

Being disabled may mean that your approach to your hobbies and passions changes, but it certainly doesn't mean a life without them! There are so many creative ways to incorporate the things that you love into your daily life, even if it's not quite in the same form as it was for your life before disability. When I became disabled, I *loved* playing the drums, something that was no longer possible when I had no movement in my legs. Although giving up my hobby was heart-wrenching, it created space for me to engage with new things, build new connections, and to incorporate new hobbies which fit so much better with my disabled life. I took up crochet and crafting, learnt new languages, adapted to archery in a wheelchair, rediscovered reading and writing, volunteered with Guide Dogs and Girl Guiding, and most recently I've become a wheelchair rugby player. Without becoming disabled, I would not have discovered so many passions which make me who I am now. My advice would be to let the grief come if it does, but to not let it close off space for discovery and exploration. At the end of the day, you never know which new interests you might discover and what new passions may be ignited!

What I learned:

- It's ok to grieve hobbies that you can no longer do due to your disability, especially if they were important to your identity. Give yourself as long as it takes.

- But there are so many great hobbies out there, and we are multi-faceted people who can be interested in several things at once. There are still so many things that you can be passionate about even with your disability – you just need to go out and find what fuels your fire!

- It's important to make space for the things we enjoy in life, the things that make us who we are, and the things that bring us those little moments of joy. Try to always make some space in your week for your hobbies for your wellbeing.

- Even with an energy-limiting condition, there are so many hobbies out there that you can participate in – find what works best for your energy or pain levels and let the joy into your life!

Reflection Time

1. Have you had to give up any hobbies because of your disability? How does this make you feel?

2. Are there any adaptive sports that you would like to try with your disability?

3. Are there any other hobbies you might like to try? How will you need to adapt them around your disability?

4. Have you researched what clubs and groups there are in your area which might be suitable for you?

Chapter 4
Maintaining Your Inner Circle
Relationships with family & friends

Over the last few chapters, we have looked at how to redefine your identity, regain your confidence, and either reclaim things you once loved or find new passions. These things can be hard enough as they are, without adding other people into the mix. The next few chapters will explore different types of relationships and how we can incorporate them into our lives as disabled people. This chapter will focus on familial relationships and friendships, whilst the next one will consider more romantic connections.

When you become disabled, it is rarely just *you* who is affected; it can have a profound impact on your close friends, family, and other loved ones. Think about how you would feel if the roles were reversed. It is incredibly difficult to watch someone you love struggling with symptoms related to their disability or grieving as they can no longer do the things that were once important to them. Your disability will hold different emotions for other people, which may spill over and affect your relationships over time. Reassessing these relationships is key to adjusting to being disabled.

Your relationships can similarly be affected if you live with an energy-limiting condition like ME/ CFS or Long-COVID. When we have limited reserves of energy, who we choose to spend our time and energies with is important. A very wise woman (otherwise known as my mum!) once told me to think of building relationships like filling a jar with marbles. Each action you or another person takes to either strengthen or harm the relationship then either adds or subtracts marbles from the jar, respectively. When you don't have a lot of energy, you want to ensure that you are spending time with people who fill up your jar with marbles. Who we choose to spend our time and energy with, then, is very telling of who is closest and most important to us.

Thinking about energy, it's certainly true that balancing our existing relationships and creating new ones will take additional energy and may increase symptoms such as pain or fatigue at first. Keeping and making friends certainly requires an effort. However, this cost is often well outweighed by the social and mental health benefits of building such connections. I do, though, recognise that not everyone will have positive relationships with family and friends. Depending on your circumstances, your birth family can be a source of great trauma, and they may be people whom you would rather forget. The great thing about becoming an adult and gaining your independence, though, is that you have the freedom to *make* your own family – what is sometimes called 'chosen family'; these are people who you select for their support, love, and respect. Just like biological families, chosen familial relationships can be incredibly important to your overall well-being. Whenever this chapter talks about familial relationships, then, please do feel free to apply it either to your biological family or to your chosen family, or both – however, you feel best fits with *your* definition of family.

Your disability will inevitably frame how you go about bolstering your existing relationships or creating new ones, perhaps within the disabled community. In this chapter, we will look at how disability intersects with losing friends, balancing current relationships, making new friends, as well as how to be a friend to someone with a disability, if you are reading this book as an ally. We shall then discuss when you might wish to disclose your disability to new friends and how to deal with unsolicited advice, so that you are well equipped to step back into your social life with a disability.

Losing friends after your disability

Let's start with the bad news straight off the bat (it does get better, I promise!): losing friends when you become disabled is unfortunately a common experience and can stem from a combination of factors. Some reasons why your friends might drift away include:

- **Awkwardness or fear of uncertainty.** Your friends may worry that they do not know how to act around you or are not sure how to handle unfamiliar situations now that you are disabled. They might avoid contact with you out of fear of doing or saying the wrong thing; this might especially be the case if your friends have never interacted much with a disabled person before. If this happens, you could try speaking to your friends about your

97

disability to demystify it for them or you could send them some resources about disability in general to help to educate them.

- **You can no longer participate in shared activities due to your disability.** Certain activities might be central to your group's dynamic and bonding, and if you're no longer able to participate in this, your friends might feel awkward or disconnected from you. You could always think of alternative activities to do instead that are accessible to you. If your friends are true friends, the activity shouldn't much matter – the main thing is that you are enjoying it together.

- **Overwhelmed by your new life.** If you have increased dependence on other people, such as your carers, friends may feel overwhelmed by the realities of your life as a disabled person. For some people, it can be a stark reminder that life can change in a split second. If this is the case, some friends might begin to withdraw from the friendship, which can be a difficult and heart-wrenching experience to go through.

- **Poor understanding of disability and internalised ableism.** Not everyone has a good understanding of disability, especially if this is something that they've not encountered much before. Poor understanding can lead to assumptions, stereotypes, and unintentional insensitive behaviour, all of which can be incredibly damaging to a friendship. Sometimes, even people who would consider themselves as supportive can hold subtle internalised ableist views, which can lead to them unconsciously distancing themselves from those with disabilities.

There are many reasons why some friendships do not last, especially once you become disabled. Sadly, this is a natural part of human life, even if it is an emotionally challenging one to experience. Losing friends can lead to social isolation and feelings of loneliness for disabled people, through no fault of their own. Disabled people can be further isolated due to the inaccessibility of social groups and places for socialising. When you become disabled at a younger age – especially if you must give up work or education – it can feel like all your peers are off enjoying life and making plans for university, graduation, travel, and new jobs whilst you are left behind.

Experiencing even more social isolation due to losing friends can take a definite toll on your mental health. So, how can you deal with losing friends when you're disabled? Firstly, I want to reiterate that it is perfectly natural for you to grieve the loss of friends, as your close relationships with others are a crucial part of who you are. However, if you're struggling with losing friends, there are several things you can try:

- **Identify your most supportive friends.** Rather than dwelling on the friends you've lost, focus instead on your more supportive ones. Think about those people in your life who actively try to understand your needs and who continue to engage with you. If you think of friendship like the marble jar we mentioned earlier,

99

these are the people you want putting marbles in your jar and vice versa.

- **Communicate openly.** Talk to your more supportive friends about your experience of losing others, about how you feel, and about how your disability might be impacting on your social life. This will help them to understand your experiences in greater depth and to better support you, as they will know what you need.

- **Find new communities.** If you're finding the loss of friends challenging, you could look for support groups for disabled people, whether in your local community or online. Talking to other people who are going through the same thing might be helpful. If you would like to build new relationships, you could look for social clubs for your hobbies or the things which interest you or even look at support groups for people with the same disability as you. Here, you can invest in new relationships with people who understand your experiences as a disabled person or who share your interests.

- **Seek professional counselling.** If you are still struggling with the emotional impact of losing a friend because of your disability, you could consider whether professional therapy might help you to process your feelings and develop coping mechanisms. Counselling can be a great option to help you become more emotionally resilient when you face difficult periods, such as losing close friends.

A final option is to **recognise that not all friendships withstand change.** Unfortunately, not all relationships are strong enough to stand up to the changes that come with disability. It might be best to accept that it's time to move on and focus instead on building new connections with others. But how do you know when it's time to let go of a friendship? Well, there are a couple of signs that things have run their course:

- **One-sided effort.** If you feel that you're constantly putting in more effort than your friend, or that you only communicate out of necessity or because you or they feel guilty, it is likely time to let the friendship fade out of your life.

- **Your friend no longer responds to important things in your life.** If something is truly important in your life, a real friend will respond, whether the answer is something you want to hear or not. If your friend is no longer responding to the important things in life, it sadly means that they're no longer prioritising you, so it might be time to move on.

- **Negative impact.** If the friendship is causing any kind of negative impact on your life - such as significant stress, anxiety, or unhappiness – it's probably time to let it go.

- **Incompatible values.** We often share values and life goals with those we are close with. If your values and goals no longer align with your friend's, it might be a sign that you are drifting apart.

- **They're not growing and evolving with you.** Friendships rarely stay stagnant as we live and change with time, but a good

101

friendship will evolve and adapt with key changes in each of your lives. If your friend is not growing and adapting alongside you, but instead remaining fixed where they are, it could be a sign that the friendship's future is under threat.

These are just a few signs that your friendship could be at risk, though you will likely know when it's time that the relationship has run its course. As difficult and heart-wrenching as it can be, sometimes it is the kindest thing to part ways amicably; it leaves both you and your former friend available to pursue the things in life which make each of you happy.

Let me tell you a little of my experience from the early days of begin disabled. I was in college, waiting for my exam results and to hopefully be accepted into a prestigious university for what – at that age – felt like the adventure of a lifetime. As my pain and other symptoms had developed slowly over the last few years, I had thought that this would give time for my college friends to acclimatise to me as a disabled person. Sadly, this did not turn out to be the case at all. It started with my friends becoming a little more distant from me, taking longer to answer my texts and not picking up the phone as frequently. When the time came to head away to university, I was so unwell that I had to take an interrupted year to get well enough to try again. Whilst I was waiting for my health to recover, my friends were enjoying the experience of being a fresher at university, with so many new clubs, activities, and new friends to get involved with. I tried to make the effort to adapt my disability around their lives, suggesting low-energy hangouts or movie nights that my body could just about manage, but the invitations were rarely taken up.

Looking back, I think that it was difficult to become disabled at that age where my friends were all trying to assert independence from their familial homes. I could no longer participate in the new activities they wished to try, and I was probably making my friends feel awkward; I was a constant reminder of how fragile their new lives really were, and how easily they could become dependent on their parents once more. With time, I slowly came to realise that the effort in the friendship was mainly one-sided. I was sending messages which stayed unread and was making calls that were never answered or returned. It came to the point that the friendship was having a negative impact on me, as I felt lonely, isolated, and left behind.

So, my then-boyfriend (now-husband) convinced me to cut ties with that group. At the time, it was incredibly hard to lose those friendships, especially as I was amidst grieving the life I could have had without disability too. Looking back with hindsight, though, I do not hold my former friends any ill will. Disability was so far out of their experience at that age, but I think they were trying to do their best with the knowledge they had at the time. Cutting ties was the best and right thing to do at that point, as trying to continue the friendship was impacting on us both in negative ways. I'm now glad that we let one another go, as it created space for me to forge new friendships when I returned to university a year later, friendships which were built on an understanding of both me and my disability.

Redefining relationships

Thankfully, losing friendships only happens in a minority of cases when you become disabled; it is much more likely that your friends will learn to adapt to your disability alongside you. If you think about it, it would be odd if your relationships did not change at all when you undergo a major life change. Your friendships or familial relationships might need changes to the way you communicate or adjustments to their overall dynamics as both you and your loved one(s) navigate new challenges and your access needs. Some relationships may strengthen due to increased dependence or support, whilst others might become strained due to these same changes. Although it can be difficult to anticipate exactly *how* your relationship might alter, there are some common ways in which relationships are redefined following a major life change:

- **Emotional impact.** Dealing with the emotional stress associated with becoming disabled – such as grief over lost identity – can impact on how you interact with other people. Your friends and family may need to be more patient and accommodating towards you, affording you empathy and understanding for exactly what you're going through. You may find that this increased support brings you and your friend or loved one closer, as you face an emotional ordeal together.

- **Communication challenges.** When one of you undergoes a major life change such as developing a disability, open and honest conversation becomes crucial in a relationship. It will help you both to express your changing needs, address any concerns, and face any changes in the relationship. If you can maintain such honest and open communication, it can bring you and your loved one much closer, helping you to feel more in-tune with one another.

- **Social life.** If you develop a disability, it's likely that your social life with your friends and loved ones will change. As we discussed in chapter three, your interests and hobbies will adapt around your disability and what you are now able to do. For instance, maybe you used to meet your friend for a run in the park before work, but you're now in a wheelchair with limited arm strength. It could be that your friend might now go for a *walk* around the park with you, rather than a run. If your friend or loved one truly cares about you, they will be more than happy to adapt around your needs if they get to spend time with you.

- **Positive impacts on a relationship.** If your disability leads to increased empathy and connection between you and your loved one, it may be that your need for support can lead to a deeper level of intimacy and closeness in a relationship. This can foster personal growth and increased resilience for you both, which can help you to navigate challenges together and strengthen the bond between you.

105

It may also lead to a greater appreciation for one another's strengths and your unique connection.

- **Unwanted impacts on a relationship.** Whilst many of the ways in which your relationships might adapt are positive, there can be some undesirable impacts of your disability upon your relationships, such as if your friend or loved one does not have a very in-depth understanding of disability and your needs. This might be quite frustrating for you, especially if they do not know much about disability and educating them becomes quite a time-consuming task.

Now that we've taken a moment to think about the ways in which developing a disability might impact on your relationships, you might be asking how on earth you both are meant to adapt to your new circumstances. Thankfully, I have a few tips which might help you and your friend or loved one to adjust to your life with a disability:

- **Acknowledge the change.** It might sound obvious, but before you and your loved one can tackle the changes in your relationship, you first need to acknowledge that these changes have occurred. Communicate openly with your friends and recognise that anyone's life circumstances can shift and that this can impact on our relationships. But, at the same time, we can weather whatever changes come with our friends and loved ones by our sides.

- **Encourage open communication.** Open communication is the ability to express your thoughts, feelings, and concerns without fear of judgement or misunderstanding. Try to foster this kind of communication with your friends and loved ones. You could then initiate a conversation with them about how you're feeling and how having a disability has impacted on your life to help them have a deeper understanding of and empathy for what you're going through.

- **Express your needs.** Whilst you're practising open communication, try to talk to your friend or loved one about your needs as a disabled person, as well as your needs in your relationship. If you clearly communicate your expectations and boundaries, it will help you both to know what to expect and will help you to be clear about how your relationship has been redefined following your disability.

- **Listen actively.** Open communication is a two-way process. Just as you would expect your friend to listen to and respect what you're saying, try to listen actively to your friend or loved one as well. Pay careful attention to their perspectives, needs, and boundaries as well, and respect them as you would wish to be respected.

- **Redefine the relationship.** If you can no longer do things which are important to you and your relationship due to your disability, you could explore alternative ways to adapt your interactions with your friend or loved one to fit the changing dynamics of the relationship. Think about other activities that you could do together, or alternative ways to socialize that still bring you both joy. If you're willing to think creatively about the issue, you'll likely come up with many other ideas on how you can redefine your relationship.

- **Be understanding.** If you or your friend are struggling to adapt to the new dynamics of your relationship after you've become disabled, try not to be too hard on yourself or one another. Acquiring a disability is a substantial adjustment to your life. Remember that everyone goes through big changes in life, and they deal with it in their own ways. Your friends may be experiencing similar life changes and trying to adapt to them as well. The best thing you can do is to be kind, empathetic, and understanding.

- **Give it time.** Sometimes, when someone goes through a big change in life – like acquiring a disability – you and your loved ones might just need a bit of quiet time and space to adjust to the new dynamics. If this happens, try to be patient with your friend or loved one. If they want to pursue your friendship, they will come back to you with time. By giving your friend the time they need, you are being empathetic and respecting their boundaries, for which they will be grateful to you.

Following a substantial life change, your relationships will continue most of the time, but they may undergo some changes to adjust to the new dynamics of your disability. You or your friend or

108

loved one might struggle with the emotional impact, the physical challenges, the changes to the way you socialise and relate to one another, or the need for greater dependence and caregiving. The best things to do in these circumstances is to give it time, be understanding, and keep open lines of communication to express your needs to your friend and reciprocate by listening to theirs. With a bit of help and patience, most relationships can survive the addition of disability to the mix!

This advice is fantastic when you're trying to keep your existing friends, but what about when you'd like to make new friends? Acquiring a disability opens so many opportunities to connect with other people and develop new friendships, especially within the disability community. So, how do you go about this?

Making new friends

A bizarre thing can happen when you become disabled, particularly if you're a mobility aid or wheelchair user. When I first started using my wheelchair, I would get so many strangers coming up to me on the street and asking if I knew their aunt's son's partner's friend who was in a wheelchair too. If I had five pounds for every time someone asked me such a question, I'd be very rich indeed by now. It's almost like non-disabled people think that disability is this weird club where we somehow all know one another. Joking aside, though, the disability community can be a fantastic place to make new friends who will have a shared perspective of what it's like to be disabled. Putting yourself out there and getting to know new people can take an enormous amount of physical and mental energy, especially if you're someone with an energy-limiting condition. But once you've found *your people*, the people who will laugh, celebrate, commiserate, and even advocate alongside you, it is a truly special bond and is more than worth the energy that it takes.

So, where are the best places to make friends when you have a disability? Some great places to make new friends – disabled or otherwise – include:

- **Local clubs, groups, and classes.** As we saw in the last chapter, these are a good place to meet new people who share your interests and who may identify in similar ways to you. Most people are now becoming increasingly aware of the need to be accessible, but if you find that the club does not meet your access needs, you could try speaking to the leader or organiser about how you can join in. For example, if you find it difficult to travel to a local group, there may be a way to make the club hybrid to allow others to attend online from their homes. You never know – you might be helping to make the club more accessible to others who were perhaps too scared to ask for help!

- **Support groups.** Hear me out, I know that support groups can be a controversial one. Some people can find support groups more of a hindrance than a benefit, especially if the conversations there take a rather negative slant. I'm also aware that support groups are not synonymous with friendship; just because you have the same disability or condition as someone else, does not mean that you'll both get on like a house on fire. But hear me out. Some people can find support groups helpful, especially if they want to get in touch with other people who have the same condition as them or shared experiences due to it. If this is what you're looking for, you could check out local in-person and web-based support groups. Often, charities linked to your disability or condition can be a good place to start. You might initially meet people through their support groups that you want to get to know better, and then a friendship can develop quite naturally from there.

- **Volunteering, work, or education.** Whether you spend your time volunteering, in education, or in employment, these can all be great places to meet new people. If you'd like to find other disabled people at your employer or institution, you could look for student groups or staff networks for people with disabilities. These can be great places to find out about the support available at your employer or place of education, and a place to meet other disabled staff members who might be able to offer their support. I actually found one of my closest friends by co-chairing our institution's network together, and who kept me going through a difficult hospital admission.

- **Social media.** If there are no clubs or groups in your area, if they aren't accessible to you, or if you struggle to leave the house, social media can be a helpful tool to allow you to connect with other

111

people, disabled or not. If you're wanting to connect with others with shared experiences, you could look for other disability or chronic-illness related accounts on your favourite social platform, or you could search for others with the same interests as you. You just need to think about the kind of hashtags people might use for this. A hashtag is a word or phrase preceded by a '#' which identifies digital content on a specific topic on social media. Once you've searched using a hashtag, you can then scroll through the posts and accounts until you find a few that resonate with you and click on them. You could always leave friendly comments on someone's posts to start the conversation!

Don't worry if you do not bond with others right away. We do not expect non-disabled people to immediately bond with every other non-disabled person they meet. The same applies for disabled people, even if we have the same disability or mobility aids or both in common! Just because you are blind or in a wheelchair, it does not mean you'll automatically get along with every other blind person or wheelchair user. Don't feel that you need to force friendships with other disabled people, especially if you have already lost friends due to your disability. Be kind to yourself and the other person and give both of you ample time to get to know one another and for a relationship to grow naturally if there is a spark there. Friendships will come with time. Just remain focused on who you feel naturally drawn towards and spend more time with them when you can – if a friendship was destined to grow there, it will.

When should I disclose my disability?

A question that often comes up when I talk to others who are disabled is when – and how – you should disclose your disability when trying to make new friends or talking to existing ones. First things first, I want you to know that you are never obliged to share about your disability, health conditions, or mental health status with anyone. You are in the driving seat and have complete control over how much or how little you want to share, how you share it, and when. However, one caveat to add is that if your disability is more easily apparent, or if you use a more visible mobility aid that gives the game away, you might have to think a bit more carefully about how you introduce your disability to others.

The second thing to know is that there's no right or wrong time to disclose your disability to potential new friends. You may wish to get it over and done with as early as possible, or you may want others to get to know you a bit better before you share this information with them. Whenever you wish to do it, it is the right time for you. Now to the question of *how* to disclose your disability. Everyone's situation is unique, but here are some things you might want to convey about your disability or health condition:

- The type of condition you have.

- How it affects your daily life?

113

- How you manage your condition.

- Your prognosis.

- How the other person can best support you.

You could see where the topic of your disability pops up naturally in the conversation or bring it up when someone asks you a question which it would be difficult to answer without mentioning it. For instance, someone might ask you what kind of things you like to do in your free time. If you have an energy-limiting condition, you could say something like: 'I used to love playing sports, but that's become a bit tricky with my disability, so now I prefer to do crafts'. This then gives the other person chance to ask more about your disability if they wish, or they could pick up on the other bits of information you have shared about yourself.

You might be worried about how someone will perceive you once you've shared about your disability. You may be concerned that they will pity you, especially if you've been through some hard times due to your disability. This is not to trivialise your experience, but one thing which can help in this circumstance is to learn to talk more light-heartedly about your disability at first, and maybe share some other information about yourself too, as in the example above. This will keep the conversation flowing and gives the other person a choice of how to continue speaking with you. You could even try making what you say a little bit humorous to help keep things light, depending on the overall tone of the conversation. This way, as the friendship develops, there will be other opportunities to talk about your disability in a more serious way, but you haven't overwhelmed the other person at the first juncture.

How do I deal with unsolicited advice?

Another question I often encounter from disabled people is how to deal with unsolicited advice, both from strangers and from friends and loved ones. Sometimes when you meet new people, or when your relationships change after becoming disabled, you can get unsolicited advice from others; this is information or recommendations that are given without you asking for them. Unsolicited advice can be difficult, as it can often come from well-intentioned friends and family who think that what they are saying is helpful, when really, we need a different kind of support from them. Most people share advice as they genuinely care and want to help us. Giving advice can also be another way that other people connect with us and show empathy. As frustrating as it can be to receive unsolicited advice, recognising these good intentions can help you to respond more compassionately.

It is worth noting, though, how continual unwanted and unsolicited advice can make us feel as disabled people. Often, the people giving the advice have not asked how we feel about a particular issue or topic, and so constant unsolicited advice can be incredibly frustrating and invalidating. It can even come across as condescending, as when we receive repeated advice, it is often about

115

something we already know or have researched a lot about, such as ways to improve our condition or possible treatments. By giving unsolicited advice, it suggests to us as disabled people that you think we are not trying hard enough to help ourselves and reveals how unaware you are of just how much of our lives are spent trying to improve or mitigate our symptoms. It can even be hurtful if your disabled friend is reaching out for emotional support, and they get unsolicited advice on what they are already doing instead. Sometimes, all we want is emotional support from our friends, not practical advice.

If you are on the receiving end of continued unsolicited advice, it can be infuriating, and you might feel that there is not much you can do to stop it. But there are some techniques you can try to fend off unsolicited advice:

- **Set limits respectfully.** Setting boundaries with your friends or loved ones may be hard at first, but it will help to set expectations for you both about the nature of your relationship. Communicate using statements from a first-person perspective, for example, 'I really appreciate your concern, but I'd prefer not to receive advice right now. I'm looking for someone who can just listen'. Be clear about your needs and respectful with what you are asking and the boundaries you're asserting. Most friends and family members will typically respond well to you asking for what you need, as they will just want to help you in any way they can.

- **Listen with an open mind.** If you do not feel able to set boundaries, try to listen to your friend's advice with an open mind. There might be a nugget of wisdom in there that could help you. Showing genuine interest and curiosity in their point of view might help to diffuse any potential tension, especially if you are finding their unsolicited advice frustrating.

- **Simply change the topic.** An alternative to setting boundaries is for you to change the topic to something more constructive. You could change the conversation to a different topic by asking redirecting questions or involving others in the discussion. Or you could take an aspect of their advice and build on it to change the direction of the conversation. For example, if your friend is suggesting you try yoga, you could ask them if they have tried any new sports or activities lately.

- **Nip it in the bud.** Another alternative is to nip unsolicited advice in the bud with a quick 'thank you'. Thank the other person for their advice but explain that you have all the medical information you need at that point in time. You can then use this to reframe the conversation and tell them what you *do* need, for instance, 'thank you, I have all the medical information I need at the moment, but what I'm really looking for is someone who can lend a sympathetic ear'.

- **Connect with others.** Sometimes, other people are not in a place themselves to give us the support we need, and that is understandable. If one of your friends or loved ones cannot support,

117

try to be empathetic – we never know what others are going through themselves. Instead, surround yourself with the type of people who *can* give you what you need in that moment.

You may have your own methods for dealing with unsolicited advice, but hopefully the examples above give you some idea of the places you could start. If you remain polite, respectful, and compassionate, most friends or loved ones will tend to respond quite well to you setting boundaries and will just be eager to help you in any way they can, even if that means not offering advice.

Being friends with a disabled person

Now that we've looked at when to disclose your disability and how to deal with unsolicited advice, you may feel more prepared when it comes to making new friends or adapting the friendships that you've already got around your disability. But what if you yourself want to befriend another disabled person with different access needs, or what if you're reading this book as an ally and want to befriend a disabled person who you've met? Internalised ableist stereotypes and misconceptions can crop up in any relationship involving disability, not just hostile ones. That's why it's so important to think consciously about how to be a good friend to (other) disabled people. Thankfully, I have some advice for you on just that!

- Keep inviting your friends to events and keep contact. Sometimes, your disabled friend might decline event invitations if

118

they have limited energy or cancel last minute if their disability and symptoms are unpredictable. Or you might find that your friend takes ages to reply to your texts or rarely feels up for speaking on the phone. You might feel that it's easier to stop texting them or stop inviting them to things, so that they don't feel that they're constantly being left out. But your disabled friend is likely to feel *more* left out if you stop inviting them to events, even if they know they cannot go. Cut your friend some slack too if they try to come but cancel on short notice, as living with a disability can be unpredictable. Trust me, most disabled people *hate* having to cancel plans or hate not being able to come at all, but we often must prioritise our health. We still like to be invited or texted, though, as it reminds us that our friends are still thinking about us. You could instead try organising flexible get-togethers or suggest accessible alternatives to support your disabled friend in being able to make it along.

- **Let your friend talk about disability.** Living with a disability can be heavy, and sometimes we just need to talk about it with our friends and loved ones. The best thing you can do is allow space for your disabled friend to discuss things and really *listen* to what they're saying. Stories of inaccessibility, discrimination, and abuse can be our daily experiences, but they might seem heavy as it feels like there is nothing you can do to help. Often, though, one of the best things you can do is just lend a sympathetic ear to your friend and believe them when they tell you about their experience, one of the most consistently grinding forms of everyday ableism is

119

when people doubt what we say or do not take our experiences seriously. Whilst you might not be able to solve any of your friend's problems, they're probably not expecting you to. Unconditional acceptance and validation will go a long way to helping them feel better.

- **Learn about their disability and disability in general.** Often, when you're from a marginalised group like disability, it always falls to you to educate others about your lived experience. This can then create the expectation that marginalised groups are *there* to educate us, which is problematic and just not true. The Internet is a great and largely free resource for us. Take the time to do some research into your friend's disability and disability issues in general as your first port of call. You could even follow disabled influencers on social media, some of whom have great resources about the realities of living with a disability. Some great influencers include: @luuudaw, @chronicallyjenni, @ninatame, @disabilitywithbailey, @disabled_eliza, @disability_visibility, @rollwithru, @jeffieplays, @katestanforth, @lucyedwardsofficial, @mollyburke, @thecatchpoles, @lucywebsterjournalist, @shelbykinsxo, @coolcrutches, @iinsidemyhead, @elliemidds, @thechroniciconic, @drhannahbarhambrown, @adisabledicon, @wheelsnoheels_, @aticcersguidetolife, @matthewandpaul, @hey_missteacher, @fashionbellee, @accessyourlifeltd, @emmaelizalines. You can still show an interest and ask your friend about their disability and their experiences, but doing your own research first will go a long way.

- **Plan inclusive activities.** When you personally don't have to worry about accessibility, it can be easy to forget about it for others. Don't be afraid to ask your friend what their access needs are, as this will help you to plan activities and get-togethers that are accessible and inclusive for them. If you're unsure about the accessibility of a place you're thinking of going, your friend will appreciate it if you do the groundwork and call ahead to check on the accessibility (you could use an app to check accessibility too – you can find out more about this in chapter ten). In other words, don't let it all fall on your friend to find accessible places and activities, but of course, you can ask for their input if you get stuck!

- **Help to advocate for your friend.** Speak up and advocate for your disabled friend where it's appropriate and where they encounter ableism. Facing ableism can be an everyday occurrence for disabled people and it can be truly exhausting to have to continually stand up for your rights and your needs. If your friend is comfortable with it, it can be a great help to them if you are willing to act as an ally and help advocate for them, as it again takes the pressure off them to continually be advocating for themselves.

- **Follow our lead on the use of humour and self-deprecation.** You might find that disabled people sometimes use dark or self-deprecating humour to lighten the mood and to help them cope with their disabilities. This can be funny for you both but

121

take extra care to read how disability jokes and humour *really* affect your friend or loved one. They may just be playing along with others so as not to make a fuss. Take the time to ask your friend how they honestly feel about it and always follow their lead about making such jokes, as not every disabled person will be comfortable with it.

I hope that the tips and advice in this chapter help you to redefine and make new friends after becoming disabled. Our relationships with our friends, family, and loved ones can be a real lifeline to support us through the ups and downs of the challenges that come with being disabled. Like anything in life, the course of friendship does not always run smooth, but I hope my advice here helps you to navigate any tricky situations as the need arises.

Whilst friendships and familial relationships can be incredibly fulfilling in our lives, many of us still yearn for something *more* – a relationship with life partner(s) with whom we can share everything in our lives. The next chapter will look at romantic relationships and how to navigate these with a disability.

What I learned:

- When you acquire a disability, it is rarely just *you* who is affected – your friends, family, and loved ones will all be impacted too.

- Disability can have either a positive or a negative impact on your relationships. Some will grow stronger, and you will become closer, whilst other relationships will fade with time.

- It's normal to grieve those relationships which don't work out but keep focused on the ones who have stayed in your life and invest in those relationships instead.

- Even if your loved ones stay by your side after you become disabled, your relationships with them will inevitably change. Communication with your loved ones is key in this situation – however hard it is, keep talking through the challenges for each of you and you will likely make it out of the other side stronger.

- You will even make new friends once you become disabled. The best thing I did was to lean into the disability community. I was soon surrounded by others who understood what I was going through and who shared my passions and interests. They're now some of my closest friends.

Reflection Time

1. Have you lost any friends because of your disability, and can you identify why this might be? How has this made you feel, and is there anything that might help you to overcome this?

2. Have any of your relationships with friends and (chosen) family changed since you became disabled? Is there anything that might help you to navigate these changes?

3. When would you feel most comfortable disclosing your disability to a new or existing friend, and why?

4. Have you faced any unsolicited advice? If you have, how did you deal with this? If not, how do you think you would best approach this if it happened?

5. If you are reading this book as a friend or ally, what steps will you take to educate yourself about your friend's disability and their experiences?

Chapter 5
Falling and Staying In Love

Romantic relationships

In the last chapter, we looked at how to approach friendships and familial relationships once you've become disabled, including making new friends and redefining your existing relationships. Let's now turn our attention to romantic relationships. Whether you believe in soulmates or not, many of us still search for another person or people with whom to share our lives and have a close relationship. Although some of the advice for platonic relationships still applies, romantic relationships also have their own unique specificities. And when you add a disability into the mix, it can present its own challenges, such as whether you make your disability evident on a dating profile, or when and how you tell prospective partner(s) about your disability. Let's look first at dating new people with a disability, before considering how to redefine existing relationships once you've become disabled.

Dating with a disability or chronic illness

Becoming disabled by no means stops you from pursuing romantic love and relationships. It is perfectly possible to date and find love with a disability, whether you're using the internet and dating apps or dating in a more 'traditional' way. But when dating with a disability, there are some things that you'll need to think carefully about:

- **Disclosing your disability**. Similarly to disclosing your disability to friends, many of the tips in the last chapter still apply to romantic relationships, but with a few additions. When it comes to your online dating profile, it's your choice whether to mention or show your disability, such as using mobility aids in profile pictures. There are benefits and drawbacks either way. On one hand, being open about your disability on your profile can help to filter out people who are not ready to be with a disabled person upfront and save time and energy whittling them down yourself. On the other hand, you might want to get to know potential partner(s) first before you disclose your disability, so that they see your personality first. Either way, it might be good to discuss your disability relatively early in the relationship, maybe after your potential partner(s) have gotten to know you on a first or second date. This will help to set expectations for the relationship and will allow you to discuss any access needs you may have for future dates. Being open and honest about your disability will help to build trust and understanding between you and your potential partner(s) too.

- **Answering your partner's questions**. If your partner(s) are looking for a long-term, committed relationship, it will be natural for them to have questions about your disability and possibly what it's like for you and others to live with. Living with and supporting another person – whether disabled or non-disabled – is a big deal.

Try not to take it too personally if your partner(s) ask questions in a clumsy or potentially insensitive way; they might really be trying to learn and be open, but this could be their first encounter with someone who is disabled. It's not your responsibility to teach them everything about disability – if they want to be with you, they ought to be willing to do some research on their own – but try to treat them compassionately if they have questions. If there is something you do not wish to share, though, you do not have to cross your boundaries. But being as open, honest, and detailed as possible with your answers will likely reassure your partner(s) and answer their questions.

- **Normalise talking about access needs.** It's not just disabled people who have access needs; we *all* have them in one form or another. If you talk openly to your prospective partner(s) about your access needs, it can help to alleviate the fear and anxiety around asking for the accommodations you need. You could even plan future dates with your partner(s), so that finding accessible places becomes a mutual responsibility and takes the burden off you as a disabled person to constantly advocate for your needs.

- **Talking about boundaries, intimacy, and sex.** Before things get heated in the bedroom, it might be helpful to discuss your boundaries around intimacy and sex with your potential partner(s). I know that this might take some of the spontaneity out of sexy time, but it will help to make it an enjoyable and safe experience for you all. Try to be open and clear with your partner(s) about what you like and need in intimate settings. This can be a more subtle way for you to introduce your access needs in the bedroom, as it means that everyone has the chance to share their needs, boundaries, and preferences.

    - **Consider any red flags you might have.** Red flags are warning signs that indicate unhealthy or manipulative behaviours, and what each of us consider to be red flags will be very personal. If you're looking for red flags connected to disability, you could see how your partner(s) treat your access needs as it will tell you a lot about how willing they *really* are to accommodate what you need and the level of care they'll offer. If your potential partner(s) only want to spend time with you in private spaces, it could be that they feel awkward being out in public with you – this is a red flag for me as it gives an indication of how confident they are to be with a disabled person publicly. If you notice any pattern in your relationship that makes you feel uncomfortable, you should consider seeking support or raising the issue with your partner(s). If they seem defensive or unreceptive, it could be that you are not as compatible as you first thought.

    This advice should hopefully help you to step out onto the dating scene. But when you have a disability, even the practicalities of planning and going out on dates can be difficult, especially if your condition causes pain and fatigue or limits the amount of energy reserves that you have. Nowadays, there are of course many ways to date that might help you in these circumstances, such as virtual or online dates. But what if you want to try to go on a date in the traditional sense of 'going out' to meet someone at the cinema, in a café, or to visit a museum or attraction? There are several things that you can do to make this kind of dating more accessible to you:

- **Agree in advance how long the date will last.** I know that this might take the spontaneity out of dating a bit, but if you and your partner(s) decide in advance how long you will spend out, it will help you to pace accordingly. If you're new to the dating scene as a disabled person, I would suggest starting small and giving yourself a buffer, so that you have a bit more time than you'll need. You'll be surprised how much energy being out with other people – and being on a date especially – will take out of you. That's why it's good to have an energy buffer, in case you accidentally go over the amount of energy you allocated to your date activities.

- **Choose a familiar location.** As you're leaving the house to go on your date, I would advise choosing somewhere close to your home that you know well. This means that you'll be familiar enough with the place you're going to; you'll know if it meets your access needs and if they can cater to any dietary requirements that you or your partner(s) might have. Choosing somewhere familiar can take some of the social stress out of the first date, as you do not have to orient yourself in a new space that could be sensorily overwhelming too. Being close to home also means that it'll take you less energy to get back home after your date. Choosing a familiar location to

129

you might mean that it is a little bit more out of the way for your partner, depending on how close you live to one another. You could always explain the reasons why you need to meet somewhere close to home, though, and you'll often find that most people will be quite accommodating once they know.

- **Make your environment more comfortable if you can.** In addition to choosing a place you already know, there may be other things that you can do to further adapt your environment to your access needs. Say you're going to a restaurant. You could research online when they have quieter periods so you can go when it's less busy, or you could discreetly ask your server to turn the background music down when you enter so it's not as overwhelming. You could ask for a quieter table, a wheelchair accessible table, or a table with plenty of light or shade when you book, depending on your disability and access needs. If you find noisier environments overwhelming, you can now buy noise-reducing ear plugs, such as Loop or Sennheiser SoundProtex, that can create a calmer environment whilst still allowing you to hear conversations. Don't worry about asking a server or restaurant manager for any adjustments that you need, as it will help you to make the most of being out with your partner(s).

- **Pace yourself.** We'll cover this in more detail in chapter eight, but pacing is essentially a strategy to manage the symptoms that come with energy-limiting conditions by balancing periods of rest and exertion. If you're going out for a length of time for a date

– even if it is something relatively low-energy like going for a coffee – consider how you can pace your day. It can help to work through in your head from the start of the date to figure out how much time and energy to expend on each activity. If you are driving or taking public transport, you might want to leave extra time in case of traffic or in case your bus or train is cancelled. This means that you won't have to expend emotional energy panicking about how you'll make it to your date. You could get ready a little earlier than you would have in the past, as well as allowing longer for your date activity, so that you can take your time and factor in rest breaks during and after your date. There are so many little ways you can pace a date to make it easier for you, so remember to check out chapter eight if you need further ideas!

- **Set your boundaries and manage expectations.** If you've got to the stage of going on physical dates with potential partner(s), it can help to speak with them about your disability and any access needs you may have. If, for example, you're choosing a location close to home, planning to take some short breaks during your date and want to spend a maximum of three hours to ensure you don't get over-fatigued, communicate that to your partner(s) so they know what to expect. You might want to set further boundaries about how your partner(s) ought to help you if needed. Many disabled people can find it quite infantilising if others just help without asking, but some are ok with this. Communicate clearly with your partner(s) about whether and how you'd like them to offer support, as it can avoid any awkward or patronising behaviour in the long run. If your partner(s) are accepting of your disability and serious about exploring a relationship with a disabled person, you should find that they're quite accepting and willing to adapt to your needs. Setting boundaries and expectations is one of the best ways to create a safe, comfortable, and accessible dating experience for everyone.

- **Have a contingency plan.** Even if you're confident that your body can manage the activities you have planned for your date, it's always a good idea to have a continency plan, as living with a disability can be unpredictable. For instance, if you have a condition that can cause fainting, seizures, or blood-sugar highs and lows, make sure you're wearing an alert bracelet and that the person you're with knows what to do in an emergency. If you have bladder or bowel issues, make sure you've taken any necessary medication before your date, that you know where the toilets are, and that you're seated close enough to make a quick dash if needed. If you can have times when speaking is too overwhelming, try to have a notes page on your phone with common phrases you can point to or invest in a set of disability communication cards. Stickman Communications, @iinsidemyhead, and the Hidden Disabilities Sunflower Scheme all have great communication cards on offer. Another option is to wear pin badges to make others aware of your disability or access needs, of which the Colourblind Zebra and other sellers on Etsy have a fantastic array. If you have an energy-limiting condition, you might have a list of 'best scenario' dates and a reserve list of 'energy-friendly dates', which include lower-energy activities like going for a coffee or seeing a film, so that you can revert to it if your main date idea is sapping your precious energy reserves too quickly. Having a disability certainly teaches you to roll with the moment!

Dating a disabled person, someone who is neurodivergent or someone with a chronic illness

So far, we've looked at how to navigate the dating scene with a disability. But what if you are supporting other partner(s) who are disabled themselves? Luckily, I have some advice about how to care for disabled partner(s) too, which comes from my own experience of being in an inter-abled relationship with my husband. If you're non-disabled – or even if you're disabled yourself – and dating a disabled partner, there's a lot you can do to better understand and show up for them. Some of these actions may take time to develop as you get to know your disabled partner(s) better, but with a bit of work and patience, they can be the foundations of a loving and long-term relationship.

- **Learn about (their) disability.** When you're disabled, it can often feel that it falls solely to you to educate the world about the realities of living with a disability and facing ableism every day. To relieve your partner(s) of this burden, take the initiative and learn about *their* disability and disability in general. You might want to learn about the main symptoms of their condition, or the impact that this has on their everyday life. You could follow influencers with the same disability or follow different influencers to learn about the spectrum of disability. You might also want to research ableism and internalised ableism and explore the disability rights movement. If you want to find out more about these topics, reading the remainder of this book is a good place to start, not to toot my own horn! Your disabled partner(s) will undoubtedly appreciate that you have taken the time to educate yourself about their experiences as a disabled person.

- **Learn about intimacy with a disability.** As well as educating yourself about your partner(s)' disability, it might help to learn more about intimacy and sexual relationships with a disability. Depending on their disability, your partner(s) may not be able to feel much in the typical erogenous zones if they have a spinal cord injury or another neurological condition but may find touch in other areas more stimulating. Your partner(s) may find certain positions painful or uncomfortable due to their disability but might be open to experimenting to find what works for you all. There is more to sex and intimacy than penetrative sex, so try to remain open to other ways of experiencing intimacy with your partner(s). Talking about intimacy with a new partner can be intimidating. Remember, you don't have to talk about everything in one go but try to talk through any anxieties or concerns with them. In doing so, you will build trust, set expectations, and assert your boundaries, laying the foundations for a safe intimate relationship. You could see this as an opportunity for you and your new partner to explore what you like and dislike together, how you might work around emotional or physical barriers, and what intimacy means for you both within the context of your relationship. As with any partner, it is important to check for consent and that your partner is happy for you to initiate physical touch and intimacy; this can be as simple as saying 'may I take your top off?' or 'would it be ok if I were to hug you?'. If you're looking for examples of sex and disability in the media, the Netflix series *Sex Education* has some great representation of disabled intimacy. Or you could consult *The Ultimate Guide to Sex and Disability: For all of us who live with disabilities, chronic pain and illness* edited by Miriam Kaufman, Cory Silverberg and Fran Odette or *Disability Intimacy: Essays on Love, Care and Desire* edited by Alice Wong.

- **Respect their needs.** Every new relationship involves learning about your partner, and what they need and want in life. Successful relationships, though, come down to whether you are prepared to meet your partner's core needs, and whether they will meet yours. Communicate openly with your partner(s) and listen attentively when they tell you what their core needs are to feel safe, emotionally and physically connected, and loved in your relationship. It may be that they need physical intimacy to feel secure, or they may need regular contact with you, or to be told that they are loved and are important to you. Whilst meeting another partner's needs is non-negotiable, *how* their needs are met is flexible and you need to make it work for you if it's to be sustainable. Part of respecting a partner's needs is figuring out how you can meet them amidst all the other demands on your time and energy in this busy modern world. Experiment and find ways that work for you to meet each other's needs and make each other feel loved, secure, and valued. Whilst you work this out, it can help if you communicate to your partner(s) that you understand their needs, why they are important to them and what your partner can expect from you going forwards.

- **Respect their boundaries.** Similarly to fulfilling their core needs, respecting a partner's boundaries is non-negotiable for a successful and healthy relationship. Not everyone feels comfortable talking about their boundaries, especially early on in a relationship. If you're not sure how your partner is feeling about a particular topic, it's best to err on the side of caution and *ask them* how they're doing; this will give you a much better gauge of how (un)comfortable they are feeling and help to establish open communication, honesty, and trust. Especially when it comes to sex and intimacy, respecting a partner's boundaries is crucial, as they may not feel comfortable with the same things that you do. It can be easy to get swept away in the moment, so it might help to try to talk to your partner about their boundaries before getting in the mood. You could set up expectations of how to communicate when things do get heated, such as how either of you will communicate if a boundary has been crossed and you want to stop. Remember as well that a partner's level of comfort and boundaries are not static but open to change; keep checking consent day-to-day, as everyone has a right to change their boundaries at any time and for any reason.

- **Talk openly about access needs.** Whilst you might let your partner(s) take the lead on what they share with you about their disability, you could encourage them to talk openly with you about their access needs and how you can best support them. If you're out with your partner(s) and see them struggling – for example, if they are a wheelchair user struggling with a curb – it's only natural to want to jump in and help them. But as we've already discussed, this can come across as patronising and can in some instances even be dangerous for the disabled person in question. Try instead to assume that they do not need help, unless they expressly ask you for support. This then gives the disabled person greater control and autonomy over their choices and when and how they seek help. It might be a good idea to check in with your partner about whether they'd like you to advocate for disabled people if you see instances of ableism, or if they would prefer to take the lead with your support. Different people will prefer different strategies, so it's worth finding out how your partner(s) prefer to tackle things.

- **Don't focus solely on their disability.** Whilst your partner's disability might be a core part of their identity and inform many of the decisions of your life together, they are so much more than their disability. See them instead as the multi-faceted and fascinating person that they are. Talk about their friends and family, their work or education, their hobbies, the sports they like playing or watching,

137

the food they like, their travels or places they'd love to go. These are only a few examples, but there is so much more to life than just their disability. Whilst your partner's disability may have an impact on their romantic or intimate relationships, try not to let it eclipse all else for you – their disability is but one piece of their identity and life.

The above advice will hopefully come in useful if you're new to dating disabled people and are looking for a few pointers to get you started in how to be intimate and how to respect your partner(s)' needs and boundaries. We've considered how to talk openly about access needs and to see your partner as more than their disability. Whilst these tips should be handy for people new to the disability dating scene, they can also be useful for people who are already in long-term relationships before disability comes along. Disabled people and their partners in this situation must first adapt to disability itself and then consider its impact on their existing romantic relationship. In what follows, we'll look at how to redefine relationships after the onset of a disability.

How to navigate an existing romantic relationship with a disability?

If you are already in a romantic relationship when you acquire or are diagnosed with a disability, this major change in life circumstances can take a significant toll on the relationship and can be particularly draining for yours and your partner(s)' emotional energy. I'm sure we all know of a few relationships which struggled when faced with the challenges that come with disability or ill health; perhaps (one of) your partner(s) had never expected to take on caring responsibilities, or they could not accept the emotional impact on their relationship. Living with a disability is hard enough as an individual, without adding the dynamics of romantic relationships into the mix.

Given the persistent stigma and misunderstanding around disability, as a disabled person you might feel frustrated that it often seems to fall on *you* to educate your friends, family, and partner(s) about disability and let them in to your life; this may especially be the case if your partner(s) have never encountered disability before and do not have much of an understanding of it. It can be tricky to adjust to your life with a disability, whilst trying to support other people who are going through this emotionally too. I say this with absolutely no judgement at all, but some relationships are just not in the right place at the time to survive this kind of emotional turmoil for all involved. If you've given the relationship your best shot, and done all you can do to make things work, but it's still draining your limited physical and emotional energy, then there is nothing wrong with cutting your losses and walking away. It's perfectly ok if your relationship(s) don't work out with disability in the mix.

Whilst this may seem a bit doom and gloom, it's worth emphasising that most established relationships *do* survive a partner becoming disabled – it will just take some adjustment on the part of each person involved and some redefining of the relationship. As well as the considerations we've already mentioned in this chapter, some of the things that you might want to discuss with your partner(s) include:

- **Maintaining open communication.** Try to talk openly about your disability and what your needs might be, as well as any concerns you have or help you might need. Remember that you're both adapting to living with your disability in your own ways, and so each of you will have their own different needs. It's ok if your partner(s) need support during this process too, as loving and supporting a disabled partner can sometimes be unbelievably hard. Maintaining communication might be difficult from time to time, but you can try to keep discussions open by encouraging feedback, being respectful of other perspectives, using multiple communication channels, and checking in with your partner(s).

- **Being patient.** Be mindful of the fact that you are adjusting to a huge change in your life, one which will bring physical, mental, and emotional changes. There will be times when you find this overwhelming or irritating, especially if you are no longer able to do the things you love independently. Encourage your partner(s) to be empathetic and imagine how they would feel in your situation, for example, if they could no longer do their favourite hobbies or activities anymore.

- **Being supportive.** One of the best things your partner(s) can do when you feel overwhelmed or frustrated is to provide encouragement and emotional support. For instance, if you are now a wheelchair user who is struggling to pursue your dream of being a successful skydiver, your partner(s) could encourage you by empathising and helping you to search for other interests or hobbies you could pick up. They might alternatively support you by researching ways that disabled people can sky dive safely, such as through tandem skydiving or specialised programmes. Or they could find activities that you could all do together, to take your mind off your worries and give you a sense of normality.

- **Avoiding over-helping.** This one may seem a bit contradictory with the advice that I've already given. Indeed, I've encouraged your partner(s) to ask you about your needs, to be supportive and help you when needed. At the same time, I would advise your partner(s) to be careful not to 'over-help'. This means doing tasks that you could quite competently do on your own without any assistance, even if it takes you longer or requires more effort to achieve them. Sometimes, doing these activities might be instrumental to your rehabilitation and physiotherapy exercises. If you can achieve tasks on your own and have not asked for support, then your partner(s) ought not jump in to help. I know it can be tempting, especially if it seems like you are struggling, but 'over-

141

helping' in this way treats disabled people as if they are fragile or vulnerable and can be quite infantilising. As a rule of thumb, if a disabled person hasn't asked for help, it's safe to assume that they don't need any support at that time.

- **Exploring intimacy.** Whilst it may take you some time to adjust to your disability, in time you may want to discuss with your partner(s) how this affects intimacy together or find ways to adapt to your needs on this front. You may want some private time and space at first to explore your own intimate and sexual relationship with a potentially altered body, sensory profile, or neurodiverse condition. Once you are comfortable with what intimacy means on your own terms, you could then explore this together with your partner(s). You might need to be open to different ways to stimulate and be intimate with one another. At the same time, try not to put pressure on yourself to perform or feel a certain way; not all intimacy needs to be sexualised. You will get back to intimacy when you are ready, even if this means that you start simple by holding hands or hugging.

- **Considering accessibility in your everyday lives.** As you adapt to your disability, you may need to take your everyday life and home environment into account, especially if your disability has altered your physical or sensory capacities. This might mean making considerable changes to your home to make it accessible for you. If you are a wheelchair user, and you have a multi-storey house, you may need to invest in a stairlift or lift. You might further have to widen doorways, make kitchen counters that you can roll under, and re-arrange furniture to allow enough space for your wheelchair to pass through. This can be overwhelming and unsettling, especially as there will be changes to your partner(s) home environment too. Encourage your partner(s) to be gentle with themselves as you navigate these changes together, as it may take them time to adapt. Try not to feel like you are on your own managing all this, too. There is plenty of support for disabled people available through most local councils, and they can help with things like grant applications to get adaptive equipment or home adaptations installed. Chapter ten has more information and tips on independent living.

As well as the above considerations, a huge thing for when you and your partner(s) are going through major life changes and redefining your relationship is to set joint goals together. There are many reasons to set goals, not least as they will help you to achieve a lasting connection with your partner(s). Sharing goals can provide a sense of direction, deepen our emotional intimacy with others, and promote open and honest communication. When you and your partner(s) understand what you are all working towards together, you are more likely to approach disagreements constructively and navigate conflict more effectively. Shared aims further build resilience, as you and your partner(s) face challenges and adapt together. Finally, joint goals ensure that partnerships are on the same page about what they want and can expect from one another, reducing misunderstandings and disappointments.

When setting goals, though, remember that relationships all look different, so what works for one might not work the same way for another. There are so many different relationship goals that you could choose to work towards, both big and small. These goals may look slightly different to the things you were aiming to achieve before you acquired your disability, and that is ok and perfectly natural. Whether you want to scale up or scale back your ambitions, it's helpful to sit down with your partner(s) and set clear and meaningful goals. But how do you go about doing this? Thankfully I've some advice for you, or you can refer to chapter ten for further guidance on setting goals:

- **Get on the same page.** The first step to setting clear goals in a relationship is to get on the same page. You need to be honest with one another about your own individual goals, and how these fit into your shared future together. Knowing what the other person or people want for the future allows you to support each other in achieving your dreams, together and as individuals. Sometimes, each partner's personal goals may seem at odds or incompatible with one another, and you may have to find creative ways to compromise and reconcile them. Alternatively, if you and your partner(s) have greatly varied visions for the future, it can sometimes be best to cool off the relationship before you come to blows.

- **Build a foundation for the future together.** Remember that your goals should encompass all parts of your relationship with your partner(s), from the way you communicate and resolve conflicts to how you support each other's personal growth and individual aspirations. You should aim to nurture emotional intimacy and cultivate mutual respect.

- **Remember that your goals are dynamic.** Your goals do not have to remain the same but can evolve alongside your relationship as it grows and changes. For instance, going out on dates might have been a priority early in your relationship, but as it develops, and you face new challenges – such as adapting to one of you becoming disabled - saving money to buy an adapted house might take more priority over date nights.

- **Set aside time each month to discuss your goals.** Incorporating goal-oriented conversations, maybe over a nice dinner, can help to build a healthy and long-lasting relationship. Be proactive in pursuing open, transparent, and honest conversations about your dreams and ambitions. Once you're in the practice of having regular discussions about it, the conversation may naturally shift to big-picture relationship goals.

- **Try to keep it fun as you trace out your future.** Having conversations about your goals in life does not always have to be so serious! Sometimes, it may feel overwhelming as you map out your future together. Instead, get excited about each other's dreams and aspirations. As overwhelming as it can be, it can also be hugely exhilarating and inspiring! Never limit yourselves and dream big!

So, you might now be asking, what kind of relationship goals can you set?

Whatever you can imagine, is probably the best answer! But if you and your partner(s) are stuck, here's some ideas you could choose to pursue:

- **Appreciate your partner's quirks and flaws**. If you become more accepting of one another's differences, it can help to deepen your bond together.

- **Be yourself within the relationship**. Encourage each other to pursue your own unique hobbies or interests and to cultivate self-love. This will not only support personal growth for each of you but will bring fresh perspectives into the relationship. Who knows, you may discover a new hobby that gets you all hooked!

- **Understand each other's love languages**. Learning each other's love languages can inform the way you connect and express affection with your partner(s). It can foster a deeper sense of understanding, appreciation, and respect for one another. Love languages can be all sorts of things from words of affirmation, giving or receiving gifts, spending quality time together, or physical touch. Find out how your partner appreciates love and try to incorporate it more into your relationship.

- **Approach conflicts and challenges as a unit**. Remember that in a relationship, you're a team. Instead of facing difficulties and challenges alone, work together with your partner(s) to find solutions to problems. You might learn to compromise and respect each other's distinct perspectives and remain supportive above all else, even when you're not on the same page.

- **Commit to communicating effectively**. Listen actively, maintain open communication, express your thoughts and feelings clearly, and remain open to your partner(s)' different perspectives.

- **Recognise when you need support**. Sometimes, we can get into the habit of always pushing on alone, rather than recognising when we might need some outside support. You and your partner(s) might learn to recognise when you all need that extra support, whether from friends, family, or trained therapists. This is crucial and shows commitment to the health of the relationship.

- **Create a judgement-free environment.** You might strive to build an environment in your relationship where you and your partner(s) all feel safe to express your thoughts, feelings, and desires without fear of judgement or criticism.

- **Make memories by spending time together**. Your relationship is likely to thrive if you and your partner(s) prioritise having fun together. Even if it's something small, like cuddling up and watching a movie together, sometimes the simplest things can make the best memories with your loved one(s).

- **Build intimacy and trust through vulnerability**. It's vital to be honest and open about your innermost thoughts and feelings with your partner(s). By the same count, it's important to be receptive when your partner(s) share what they are thinking and feeling.

- **Prioritise each other every day**. If you regularly show that your partner(s) are your priority through your actions and your words, you're well on your way to building the foundations of a strong and lasting relationship. Prioritising each other could mean taking time for one another, being present during conversations, using your partner's love language, or doing small acts of kindness for your partner(s).

Finally, here are some questions that you and your partner(s) could use during your goal-oriented conversations:

- Where do you want to be in a year/ at the end of the year?
- What do we want to have done as partners by the end of the year?
- Where do we want our relationship to be by the end of the year?
- What financial goals do you want to set?
- What health and wellbeing goals do you want to set?
- How are we going to prioritise our relationship with one another this year?

148

- How do you want to grow personally / are there any goals I can support you with this year?
- What core memories do we want to make together this year?
- Are there any projects around the house that you want to work on this year?
- Are there any travel trips we want to make this year?

Romantic relationships form an important part of our lives, providing us with comfort, support, and love. If you're seeking a new relationship or are already in an established one, disability can have an incredible impact upon it, especially as your partner(s) learn to adapt to this new dynamic in their life too. I have been in an inter-abled relationship since I was around seventeen which, as you may remember, was around the time when I first became disabled. When it became clear that I would have a life-long disability, I gave my partner the option to leave the relationship without judgement. But he refused because my personality and who I was as a person mattered more to him. This meant that we had to have some very frank conversations early on in our relationship about how things would work around my disability.

Since then, we have faced our fair share of challenges, and the course of our relationship has not always run smoothly. My partner found it difficult to see me struggling with symptoms or tasks which were now difficult due to my disability; his instinct was often to jump in and offer support, but he had to gradually relearn this response as he understood that maintaining my independence was important to me. The biggest challenge we had to face came in our early thirties, when I developed a life-threatening pulmonary embolism and was hospitalised on a high dependency ward for several weeks. Throughout the scariest time of our lives thus far, my partner and I remained strong together, loving and supporting one another through the tears, tests, and treatments. Due to these frequent emergencies, my partner has experienced a lot of generalised anxiety around my disability and its impact on our lives, so we sought out professional counselling for him to discuss his concerns. Trusting me has helped to alleviate some of this anxiety too. My partner trusted that I knew my body and that I would tell him if I felt something wasn't right or if something serious was going on. He is my soulmate and amber warning light for when I need to take things easier.

We therefore found that communication and mutual respect for what each of us brought to the table were especially important in our inter-abled relationships. Open and honest communication enabled us to work through any issues as they arose, and to let each other in on how we were feeling. Our main advice for managing relationships with disability in the picture would be to: maintain open communication with your partner(s); be patient with them as they navigate life with a disability; respect their boundaries; support them with their needs, without over-helping; and (re-)explore what intimacy means to you together. A final key piece of advice is to share your goals with your partner(s). Do you want to get married, have kids, or buy a house? Sometimes your disability might mean that these traditional life goals happen on a different time scale, or even not at all; your goals may change after acquiring a disability – or they might not! Either way is perfectly ok, as it's up to you and your partner(s) to define what your relationship and life together will be!

What I learned:

- Dating with a disability poses its own challenges, but it's by no means impossible!

- You'll have to make some key decisions about how and when you disclose your disability to potential partner(s). Hard as it may be, disclosing your disability is a good litmus test of which partner(s) aren't serious about being with a disabled person and which one(s) will stick around.

- We all have access needs and boundaries when it comes to intimacy and sex. Normalise talking about yours and your partner(s)' to take the anxiety out of intimate encounters.

- If you want to date someone with a disability, put in the groundwork. Learn a bit about (their) disability, consider their needs when being intimate, talk openly about access requirements and always look to the person they are beyond their disability.

- When you're already with someone, and one of you becomes disabled, it is only natural that your disability will have an impact on your relationship and your partner(s)' lives. Maintaining communication and being patient with one another as you settle into the new status quo is key to weathering the challenges posed by disability.

- As a couple, you are investing in a life shared together. Never stop setting goals for what you want to achieve together.

Reflection Time:

1. When would you feel most comfortable disclosing your disability to potential partner(s) and why?

2. What steps will you take to make your dates accessible for your needs? What will be your contingency plan?

3. How might you go about normalising talking about access needs with your partner(s)?

4. If you're reading this book as a friend or ally, or want to date another disabled person, what steps will you take to learn about your partner(s)' disability and their access needs?

5. If you're disabled and already in a relationship, think about how you and your partner(s) will work through adjusting to life with a disability together.

6. How will you talk about setting goals with your partner(s)? Are there any other goals that you might want to set together?

Chapter 6
Which Way Now?

Education, employment, and benefits

Thinking about the other components which make up our lives and identities, education and employment often take up a large amount of our time. Whilst some disabled people cannot work or study at all, many do enter education or employment in some capacity and find fulfilling roles. But navigating these fields with a disability does present its own challenges. What are your rights as a disabled person in education or employment? How do you access support for your disability? What options are there if you are no longer able to work? These are just some of the questions that this chapter hopes to answer. We will talk about further and higher education and employment in the UK, looking at what your rights are, what you can expect, and how to access the support that you need. Let's start with education, and later we'll move on to employment.

Further and higher education in the UK

Further and higher education can be an exciting, stimulating, and formative time in our lives if it's what we choose to pursue. But what if you're a disabled student? Under the Equality Act 2010, it's against the law for schools or further and higher education providers to treat students unfavourably due to their disability. This includes:

- **Direct discrimination.** This might be refusing to allow a student to study there or excluding them from educational activities.

- **Indirect discrimination.** This might include only providing application forms in one format, which may be inaccessible to students with certain access needs, thereby excluding them.

- **Discrimination arising from disability.** This might mean a college or university prevents a student from taking a course due to their disability.

- **Harassment.** Harassment might include a lecturer shouting at a student for not paying enough attention, when their disability prevents them from easily concentrating.

- **Victimisation.** Victimisation might take the form of a college or university excluding a disabled student for complaining about harassment.

In addition to not treating disabled students unfavourably, education providers in the UK must make 'reasonable adjustments' to ensure that students are not discriminated against or disadvantaged due to their disability. Reasonable adjustments could include offering additional learning support, assistive technologies, extra time in examinations, or aids to help you study and succeed. Further and higher education institutions must ensure that their buildings are accessible to disabled students. They should have a designated person in charge of disability issues, who you can talk to

154

about the support that they can offer you. Outside of your education institution, you can ask your local social services for an assessment to help with your day-to-day living needs if, for example, you need help living independently at university.

More about reasonable adjustments

As we've already noted, colleges and universities have a legal duty to try to remove the barriers that you face in education due to your disability. This is called making reasonable adjustments. To have a legal right to such adjustments, you need to be defined as disabled under the Equality Act 2010. This will depend on *how* your disability affects you, rather than what condition or diagnosis you have. The Act defines a disability as 'a physical or mental impairment that has a substantial and long-term negative effect on someone's ability to do normal daily activities'.[10] You therefore do not need to have a formal diagnosis to meet the legal definition of disability in the UK. This is incredibly helpful, especially due to the long waiting times to be diagnosed for certain conditions, such as ADHD and autism. If you think you might be neurodivergent, for instance, most UK universities will not insist on a formal diagnosis

---

[10] UK Government, (2010) Definition of disability under the Equality Act 2010 [Online]. Available at https://www.gov.uk/definition-of-disability-under-equality-act-2010 (Accessed 8 August 2025).

before offering learning support or making reasonable adjustments to help you with your studies.

But what kind of reasonable adjustments might you be entitled to? There are all kinds of adjustments that can be considered 'reasonable'. They might be things such as getting lecture notes and slides in advance; receiving learning resources in alternative formats (e.g., large print or braille); getting adaptive equipment or aids; having BSL interpreters or scribes; using specialist computer software; accessible teaching rooms; or accessible student accommodation. You might be able to access reasonable adjustments for assessments and examinations, too, such as taking your exam in a smaller room with no other students, having comfort breaks, receiving additional time, or dictating or typing your answers instead of handwriting them. You can find some examples of typical adjustments that people request, broken down by disability, in the following pages.

There is no set definition of what is 'reasonable' in the Equality Act 2010. What is deemed 'reasonable' will depend on other factors such as cost, practicality, effectiveness, disruption to others, and health and safety. The best approach is to work with your university or college to find adjustments that are considered both 'reasonable' and which meet your access needs. If your college or university deems something 'unreasonable', they should try to help you find acceptable alternatives. Alternatively, you could approach local disability charities, support groups, or online forums to help you to find alternatives that you can suggest to your institution.

To set up reasonable adjustments, you'll need to find out who supports disabled students at your university or college. They might be called something like the 'Disability Support Service' or 'Disabled Students' Service'. These services have disability advisors who can support you in implementing the reasonable adjustments that you need and making your tutors aware of your access needs. In some instances, they can help to speak to or advocate for you with your tutors. My advice would be to speak openly with your disability advisor about the challenges you're facing due to your disability, what you need, and what kind of adjustments that you think will help. If you have not already had a needs assessment for your disability at college or university, ask your advisor for one as they can often carry this out. This assessment will then give you a report telling you what equipment, support, and adjustments you might need. Some adjustments can take time to put in place, especially for exams and assessments. I'd advise asking your disability advisor to get this started as soon as possible, either at the start of a new term or academic year. If you already know what adjustments you need, you might even be able to ask them to be put in place *before* the start of term. And it's always worth checking with your advisor that your adjustments are definitely in place *before* the start of the assessment and exam season!

157

Once you've met with your disability advisor, you will often get a letter or report in writing to confirm what you talked about, what happens next, what your advisor needs to action, and what reasonable adjustments were agreed in the meeting. Your advisor might then encourage you to apply for a Disabled Student's Allowance (DSA) to get a more in-depth needs assessment and to pay towards certain adjustments (more on this later in this chapter). Your disability advisor is the best place to go to for getting support for your condition. However, if they are unavailable, you might want to try the Students' Union (SU) welfare officer, Disability Rights UK student helpline, or the Equality Advisory Support Service helpline to get support with implementing reasonable adjustments for your studies.

Examples of reasonable adjustments by condition
ADHD & Autism:

- A dedicated support worker.

- For staff to have awareness training.

- Specialist tuition support.

- Extra time in exams and automatic extensions for assessments.

- Allowing students to present their work to academic staff or to make a video presentation instead of written assignments.

- Support worker or alternative ways to complete group work.

- Use of a prompter to keep focused in exams.

- Buddy system with peers.

- A quiet room for sensory overwhelm.

- Extensions on library loans.

Blind or partially sighted:

- A mobility trainer to learn key routes around campus.

- Drawing up a Personal Emergency Evacuation Plan, or PEEP – this is a personalized plan for anyone who might need assistance during an emergency evacuation, such as those with a disability.

- Support worker or sighted guide.

- Support of a Guide Dog.

- Scribes, amanuenses, or note takers for lectures or exams.

- Large print or Braille transcription services.

- Access to lecture recordings to listen back to them.

- Alternative arrangements for placements for field work.

- Use of assistive technology in exams.

- Extended library loans and special arrangements for photocopying.

- Additional time in exams.

- Automatic extensions on deadlines when needed.

- Assistive software to allow you to participate in class activities.

d/Deaf or hard of hearing:

- Sign language interpreter or lip-speaker.
- Note-takers.
- Induction loop systems in lecture theatres and classrooms for hearing aids.
- Drawing up a Personal Emergency Evacuation Plan, or PEEP.
- Textphone at home or at least somewhere accessible on campus.
- For staff to receive d/Deaf awareness training.
- For people you spend a lot of time with to have access to BSL classes, if they wish.
- Flashing light or vibrating pad system for the fire alarm in student accommodation.
- For materials in video format to be captioned.

Medical conditions:

- Alternative arrangements for work and deadlines.
- Timetable planning to avoid fatigue.
- Having a rest room on campus to minimise fatigue.

- Medical support for emergencies.

- The opportunity to intermit studies and contact with staff during any periods away from study.

- Supplying notes or arranging catch-up sessions if you miss lectures due to your condition.

- Specialist adapted computer equipment.

- Extra time and rest breaks in examinations and automatic extensions to assessment deadlines.

- Extensions on library loans.

- Ergonomic furniture to manage chronic pain.

Mental health conditions:

- Timetable planning.

- Help with your work to manage stress.

- Access to mentoring and study skills support.

- Support from welfare and counselling staff.

- Extensions on library loans.

- A named contact for you to go to if you need support.

- Computer equipment and specialist software to enable you to study at home.

- A quiet room on campus to rest in.

- Extra time and rest breaks in examinations.

- A prompter to keep you focused during examinations.

161

Physical disabilities/ mobility problems:

- Physically accessible classrooms.

- Timetable planning to ensure accessibility.

- Personal assistants or mobility helpers.

- Adapted furniture to help you to study at home.

- Powered wheelchair or mobility scooter and facilities to charge it.

- Assistive technology to help you to study.

- Typing or transcription services.

- Digital recorders or scribes for lectures.

- Support for any practical work and fieldwork on your course.

- A rest room on campus to help with fatigue.

- Extra time for coursework and examinations.

- Drawing up a Personal Emergency Evacuation Plan, or PEEP.

Specific learning difficulties, such as dyslexia or dyspraxia:

- Specialist tuition support.

- Use of assistive technology in examinations.

- Handouts and reading lists in advance.

- Special photocopying arrangements.

- Extra time to read, understand and prepare answers.

162

- Oral examinations in addition or in place of written examinations.

In addition to the reasonable adjustments discussed above, there are other kinds of support available for disabled students in the UK. Let's take a closer look.

Disabled Students' Allowances (DSA)[11]

Disabled Students' Allowances (DSA) are a grant that can help you to meet disability-related costs that you incur whilst studying at university. In England, the maximum allowance is currently around £27,000 per year, excluding disability-related travel costs, on which there is no cap. DSAs are available for both full-time and part-time undergraduate and postgraduate students, and are not means-tested. This means that neither your income nor your parents' or guardians' incomes are considered when assessing how much DSA you ought to receive. Previous periods of study do not affect your eligibility for DSA either.

DSA does not fund items or costs related to your disability that you would have regardless of whether you are studying or not. It does not cover costs that non-disabled students would have to pay.

---

[11] Please note that all information was correct at time of publication [31 October 2025]. Please always check Government websites for the most up-to-date information in cases of changes to this scheme.

This is why – if you are recommended specialised IT equipment under DSA – there is currently a £200 contribution you need to pay towards this, as most students would expect to buy a basic laptop or tablet for their studies nowadays.

In England, you can apply for DSAs at the same time as you are making your main funding application to Student Finance England (SFE). You can even apply before you have a confirmed place at college or university, so that you can get your support in place by the time you start your course. Some types of support may require extra funding through DSAs, and you may need a specialist assessment. If you have a specific learning disability, you will also need a specialist assessment when applying for DSAs to help determine the type of support you will need. The costs of such assessments are usually covered in your DSA award.

For more information on Disabled Students' Allowances, you can check out the DSA webpage on gov.uk.

Charities and grants[12]

DSAs are great to help you access support, but sometimes they are not enough, or they will not cover the specific disability-related costs you have, such as specialist accommodation. Thankfully, there

---

[12] Please note that all information was correct at time of publication [31 October 2025]. Please always check each charity's website for the most up-to-date information in cases of changes to this scheme.

are plenty of grants and charities out there who want to help disabled students thrive and succeed at university or college. Each will have their own eligibility criteria, so check carefully whether you qualify and what you need to do to apply.

But how can you find these grants? A good old web search can come in handy here, but there are some sites dedicated to listing grants that students can apply for:

- Turn2Us: https://grants-search.turn2us.org.uk/
- Disability Rights UK: https://www.disability-grants.org/higher-education-grants.html

The **Snowdon Trust** is another charitable organisation who seek to help disabled students thrive in the UK. Their grants help to remove barriers by funding disability-related study costs, so that disabled students can access and participate fully in their studies in higher education. The Trust can help to step in where DSAs might not cover disability-related costs, and they have two types of assistance available. The Snowdon Trust have grants that you can apply for to cover things like specialist equipment, assistive technology and software, mobility equipment, the additional cost of accommodation, note-takers, and other vital human support. They also have a Master's Scholarship scheme, which aims to accelerate the most exceptional disabled students through their master's level studies and into leadership roles in all their forms. These students should be visible role models and spearhead disability inclusion as the influencers of the future. For former scholars and grant holders,

165

the Snowdon Trust runs the Disabled Leaders' Network in conjunction with the Global Disability Innovation Hub at UCL.

Disabled Students' and Disability Inclusion Services

Most UK universities now have services for disabled students which work towards disability equity and inclusion in higher education. Each service, made up of disability advisors, is a place where disabled students can come to discuss the difficulties that they are having with their studies and the types of support that can be put in place. In addition to agreeing reasonable adjustments, disabled students' services can support DSA, grant, or benefit applications or may even have their own support fund for students struggling with disability-related costs. You may even be assigned an advisor who can check in on you, and whom you can approach if you are having any problems or challenges. If you do not wish to approach the disabled students' service at your institution, many universities now have dedicated Equity, Diversity, and Inclusion (EDI) teams, who can help with any disability-related issues you may be facing. It's worth checking to see what the arrangements are at your university so that you know who you can go to if you need support.

Funding for personal care[13]

Personal care or assistance is the practical support that you need to live your daily life independently. This is rarely covered by DSA or other higher education grant funding but can be essential in supporting a disabled student to live away from their typical home environment on their own. There is support you can access to help you with living independently. Under the Children and Families Act 2014, young disabled students with education, health, or social care requirements can ask for an assessment of their needs. Local authorities in England must carry out the assessment and prepare an Education, Health, and Care (EHC) plan for those who need one. If you have an EHC plan, you can request a personal budget. This will give you greater choice and control about how you buy your support, how you employ personal assistants whilst studying, and who you choose to provide this service to you. Whilst this may come with its own challenges – such as re-arranging your own care rota if one of your carers is off sick one day – it can create so many opportunities for young disabled people to live independently who otherwise might not be able to.

---

[13] Please note that all information was correct at time of publication [31 October 2025]. Please always check Government websites for the most up-to-date information in cases of changes to this scheme.

My experience in Higher Education

My first experience of Higher Education happened as I was just becoming disabled. I had only been at university for a few weeks, which had mostly been spent in and out of hospitals, and so I decided to interrupt my studies for a year whilst I underwent investigations. During that year, I was diagnosed with various conditions and decided to swap to a university closer to home for continuity of my medical care. Whilst it was initially very hard to accept interrupting my studies after I had worked so hard to get to university, this year allowed me to get the right kind of support in place that would give me the best chance for my second attempt at university a year later. I connected with the disability service at my new institution and met with an advisor to discuss my needs and the support they could offer.

When I began my second attempt at university, my mobility was slowly deteriorating, and I needed help to get around the large city campus that I had chosen. Thankfully, my university's disability service was able to lend me a mobility scooter, which was instrumental in enabling me to get around the campus before I could acquire my own mobility aid to help. That said, it certainly took me a moment to learn how to handle the mobility scooter, especially after I accidentally drove my mum into a bin on our first outing! Small accidents aside, the scooter gave me an incredible amount of independence, not just to access my studies, but to live independently and to participate in the more social aspects of university life with my peers. Connecting with the university's disability service helped me in many other ways too. My advisor set up several reasonable adjustments to support me, such as extended library loans, automatic extensions to assignment deadlines, access to a rest room on campus, and extra time and rest breaks in examinations, to name but a few. My advisor helped to convey my access information to my university lecturers, so that they were aware of how they could support me in class. It was this support which enabled me to become a high achiever at university.

Reasonable adjustments weren't the only support I was able to access at university, though. As someone who had been newly diagnosed during the year I interrupted, it was tough navigating a whole new world of access needs and disability support. This was why my disability advisor at the university encouraged me to apply for a Disabled Student's Allowance (DSA). I had a rough idea of the type of support I *might* need, but after having my assessment, I had a much clearer picture of what the DSA could offer. DSA provided a specialist lightweight tablet laptop and specialist software so that I could carry a laptop to lectures without straining my joints and the software helped when I was feeling fatigued but still needed to do university work. When I entered my PhD studies, the DSA funded taxis to and from university for me, as I was finding it hard to utilise public transport with my pain and fatigue. Without their support, I would not have been able to access my studies as easily as I did.

Whilst the DSA supplied me with a lot of the things that I needed to succeed, I still needed more support than they could offer. Due to a mast cell condition, I reacted extremely badly to perfumes and household cleaners and so needed my own self-contained and wheelchair-accessible flat - rather than shared university halls - which came at a much higher cost. On the advice of my DSA advisor, I applied to the Snowdon Trust for a grant to help with the additional cost of accessible accommodation. I was incredibly lucky to receive their support and so was able to stay in safe and accessible accommodation throughout my degree. This not only supported me to succeed in my studies but enabled me to live independently for the first time, just like my peers. It was due to the Snowdon Trust's support that I was able to feel like any other university student, living away from home and gaining my independence.

Getting the right support at university wasn't always straightforward and it took a fair amount of perseverance. But, in the end, it was worth it. Through all these sources of support combined – from my university disability service to the DSA, and the Snowdon Trust – I was able to get the support that I needed to thrive at all aspects of university life. For other students, I would encourage you to keep advocating for your needs and don't be reticent about applying to all the different sources of support and funding that you can. You know your access needs best, so have faith in your instinct and be tenacious in going out and getting what you need.

There is a lot of support out there as a disabled student to enable you to make the most out of your university or college studies. Sometimes, though, you will need to be proactive to search for the support that will work best for you. It can feel frustrating that the onus is constantly put on you as a disabled person to fight for what you need. In an ideal world, university and college study would be accessible to disabled students without us having to be assertive about our access needs. Sadly, we aren't there yet. But there is support available out there, so my advice would be to grab it by the horns. University or college can be a thrilling adventure. It can expand your horizons and open you up to a plethora of opportunities during your course and after you've graduated. With recent improvements in support for disabled students, your disability is certainly not something that will hold you back from thriving at university.

Your rights in employment in the UK

Having looked at university and college study, you might be asking what happens once you've graduated and entered the world of work. Or maybe you chose not to go to university and to enter the workforce earlier. The good news is that there is plenty of support out there for disabled employees. Under the Equality Act 2010, it is illegal for employers to discriminate against you due to your disability. This covers all aspects of the employment process, including application forms, interview arrangements, job offers, terms of employment including pay, promotion or training opportunities, and dismissal or redundancy. You cannot be chosen for redundancy because you are disabled, nor can your employer force you to retire if you become disabled.

When an employer is recruiting, they can make limited enquiries about your health or disability. This might help them decide if you can carry out tasks which are essential to the job, or if the interviewers need to make reasonable adjustments to help you, or if the employer wants to increase the quantity of disabled people on their work force. We'll discuss about how and when to disclose your disability to an employer shortly.

As in the education sector, employers must make 'reasonable adjustments' to prevent you from being disadvantaged compared to your non-disabled colleagues in the workplace. Reasonable adjustments could mean modifications to your working hours or providing you with a specialist piece of equipment that assists you in doing your job. If you feel that you need reasonable adjustments, you're best speaking to your line manager or HR representative about the support you think you might need. They will be able to advise whether it is reasonable compared to the business' needs, and how and when your support can be put in place. There are also other ways to access the support you need, such as through Access to Work, which we will discuss later in this chapter too.

There are so many advantages for employers to hire disabled people. Studies show that disabled people make valuable and reliable employees, and that they tend to be less likely to leave an employer than their non-disabled colleagues.[14] This can lead to increased productivity within the workforce. Due to their loyalty, disabled employees can reduce staff turnover and thereby save on the cost of recruiting to replace employees who have moved on. Hiring disabled people can further improve morale through being an inclusive workplace which supports people with disabilities. Whilst some argue that employing disabled people is expensive due to the accommodations they need, most adjustments typically cost very little at around £75 per person on average.[15] With all these benefits, it certainly pays off for companies to be inclusive and accessible for the skilled talent pool of disabled employees, otherwise they're missing out!

How and when to disclose your disability to an employer

There are several moments in the process of acquiring a job when you could disclose your disability to an employer. There is no right or wrong answer here, as it is up to you when and how you wish to disclose this information about yourself. You could declare

---

[14] Mencap. (2023) Fact sheet 2: The benefits of hiring someone with a learning disability in your workplace [Online]. Available at https://www.mencap.org.uk/resource/fact-sheet-2-benefits-hiring-someone-learning-disability-your-workplace (Accessed 8 August 2025).

[15] Business Disability Forum. (11 September 2024) Reasonable adjustments – what are they and why are they important [Online]. Available at https://businessdisabilityforum.org.uk/resource/reasonable-adjustments-smes/ (Accessed 8 August 2025).

your disability during the application process, such as in your application form or covering letter. Alternatively, you could disclose your disability before the interview – this is a good idea if you feel that you need any reasonable adjustments to help you to perform your best. You could even mention your disability during the interview itself and discuss it in a positive way, or give examples of how you have managed challenges associated with your disability and the skills you've developed as a result. You might instead want to wait to disclose your disability until after you've received the job offer, or during your employment itself. You can discuss your disability if your condition changes or if you need additional reasonable adjustments. You might wish to disclose your disability to your employer if:

- Your condition starts affecting you more than it used to, and you need more support.

- You're moving to a new role and need your support to continue.

- You receive a new diagnosis.

- You need specialist equipment for your disability.

There are pros and cons of disclosing your disability both early and later in the application and onboarding process. If you disclose your disability early on, it gives your (potential) employer more time to implement any reasonable adjustments you might need, so that you can hit the ground running when you start your new job. If you disclose your disability later in the process, your employer may find it harder to put your adjustments in place in time. But this approach does give you more time to get to know the people around you and to build up trust before you disclose your disability. It is completely up to you, depending on what you feel most comfortable and confident with, and on what will give you the best chance to shine at interview and secure the job.

If you do not wish to disclose your disability during the application process, it might still be helpful to discuss it with your employer once you have been offered the position. This will help them to put in place any reasonable adjustments that you may need, as well as triggering things like Access to Work if you need additional support. If your disability is more visible – for example, if you use mobility aids or if you need reasonable adjustments for the interview or tests – it may be better to disclose your disability at an earlier stage, such as on the application form. Not only will this avoid any surprises for your potential employer, but it will also afford you the best and most accessible application process possible, giving you the best chance of securing the job.

Sometimes, some people are concerned about disclosing their disability to an employer as they fear discrimination, stigma, or exclusion. These are valid concerns and, historically, disabled people have faced discrimination in the workplace. Things have changed over the last half-century, though, with the rise of the disability rights movement around the 1970s, and there are now many benefits to disclosing your disability. For one, it helps employers to create more diverse workforces, where disabled voices are represented. If you do declare your disability to an employer, they then have a legal responsibility to support you and to ensure you do not face discrimination due to your disability. Employers should provide reasonable adjustments, they should not ask you to 'prove' your disability to access support, and they should create an environment where employees feel safe and comfortable to talk about disability. At the end of the day, your employer can only provide adjustments if they know about your disability and how to best support you.

This was certainly my experience with my current employer. At first, I had been worried about declaring my disability. As a full-time wheelchair user with other access needs and multiple rare conditions, I was concerned how they would feel about having me on the team. So as not to cause any surprises for the interviewers, I declared my disability when I was invited to interview. This was so that they could ensure the interview room was wheelchair accessible. I was so nervous when the day of the interview arrived. Due to the Covid-19 pandemic, I had only ever done job interviews online before, so I was not sure what to expect from this face-to-face encounter.

But the experience was incredible! The building that my interview was in was wheelchair accessible, it had a lift, and it had both a right-hand *and* a left-hand transfer disabled toilet. What a luxury! The interviewers had made sure that all my reasonable adjustments were in place, which instantly made me feel at ease and able to focus on doing my best at the interview. I knew instantly that I really wanted the job and to work there. It was clearly a place where disabled colleagues were valued. Thankfully, I received a call offering me the position that very afternoon, and I've remained there ever since!

After being offered the position, I was glad that I had already declared my disability. Before I started, I got to meet with my line manager, and we discussed my access needs and the reasonable adjustments I needed in more depth. They then made sure that all these adjustments were in place *on the first day* of my employment, which felt truly incredible. It meant that I could just come in and focus on learning the job at hand, rather than worrying that I would need to advocate for myself to get the support I needed. Declaring my disability early in the process also helped my employer to trigger things like Access to Work to apply for funding for any specialist equipment that I needed. Overall, I would certainly recommend disclosing your disability to your employer relatively early in the process. Not only will it give you the best chance to succeed, but it will help you to gain a sense of the employer, how they treat disabled colleagues, and whether you would like to work for them. It will also give your potential employer the best chance to implement any reasonable adjustments that you need prior to your start date, allowing you to focus on doing the job you applied for.

If you disclose your disability, your employer can support you by putting reasonable adjustments in place, but there are other kinds of support available for disabled employees too. Three of the main ones are Access to Work, the Disability Confident Scheme, and the Business Disability Forum. Let us look at all three in turn.

Access to Work[16]

Access to Work is a publicly funded government grant scheme in the UK which helps disabled employees by providing practical and financial support. For example, Access to Work might help to pay for a BSL interpreter or lip speaker to work with you if you are d/Deaf or hard of hearing and need communication support. There are currently some proposed changes to the kinds of support that the Access to Work scheme can provide.[17] However, these need to undergo further parliamentary debate, whilst disabled people's organisations (DPOs) are opposing these changes and advocating

---

[16] Please note that all information was correct at time of publication [31 October 2025]. Please always check Government websites for the most up-to-date information in cases of changes to this scheme.

[17] Please note that all information was correct at time of publication [31 October 2025]. Please always check Government websites for the most up-to-date information in cases of changes to this scheme.

instead for a reform that focuses on genuine employment support for disabled people rather than cost-cutting.

At present, to be eligible for Access to Work, you must be 16 or over, be in or about to start paid work, and have a condition that affects your ability to do your job or travel to work. Your employer cannot apply for Access to Work for you, so you will need to do this yourself. You can similarly apply for it if you are self-employed, as any kind of paid work is valid, provided that it is above the lower earnings limit. Crucially, you do *not* need a formal diagnosis to apply for Access to Work, but it helps if you can explain your access needs on your application. This is especially helpful when there are long waiting times for specialists and diagnoses.

Access to Work can only assess you once you have a written job offer. But you can apply for it up to 6 weeks before you start work, or within 1 month of starting work, and your application will be expedited. If you are already in work and need support, you can still apply for Access to Work, but it will likely take longer for your application to be processed. You do not need to receive disability benefits to apply for Access to Work, nor does it affect any benefits that you already get.

It's important to note that Access to Work is a grant and the funding does not need to be paid back. Once you have received your support, you have up to 9 months to claim your Access to Work grant. If your condition or your job changes, you can contact the Access to Work team for a review. They will typically review your circumstances or support needs after a set period, or if your circumstances change. They usually contact you up to 12 weeks before your support is due to end and, if you would like to continue, then you will need to renew your grant.

Whilst Access to Work is a useful scheme to help disabled employees get the support that they need in employment, there are some things which it cannot fund. These include:

- Reasonable adjustments that your employer must make under the Equality Act 2010.

- Support that you and your employer put in place before you applied for Access to Work.

- Equipment that is standard for the job you do.

- Getting a diagnosis, such as paying for a dyslexia or ADHD assessment.

Access to Work is great if you need specialist equipment or financial support which your employer cannot provide. For me, it was instrumental in getting the wheelchair I needed to be able to get to, from, and around my workplace easily. I wouldn't be where I am in my career without their support. My main advice would be to apply as early as you can once you know the type of support you might need, as if you apply before you start your job, your application will be expedited. Otherwise, there can be relatively long wait times.

The Disability Confident Scheme[18]

To give some context on how widespread disability is, there are nearly 6 million people of working age in the UK who are disabled or who have a chronic health condition. This amounts to approximately 19% of the UK population. There has, however, historically been a substantial gap between the number of disabled people versus non-disabled people in employment. There are several reasons why this might be, including various jobs being inaccessible to people with disabilities. To help counter these statistics, Disability Confident is a government scheme which encourages employers to recruit and retain disabled talent by providing them with free guidance and resources.

The Disability Confident scheme helps employers to draw from the widest pools of jobseekers, including securing skilled, loyal, and hardworking staff, thereby reducing employee turnover. Importantly, employers who are part of the Disability Confident scheme must ensure that disabled candidates receive an interview if they meet the essential criteria for the job, and so it ensures that disabled people have an increased chance of securing a job in the first place. Through the Disability Confident scheme, many employers are challenging attitudes towards disability, increasing

---

[18] Please note that all information was correct at time of publication [31 October 2025]. Please always check the Disability Confident Scheme's website for the most up-to-date information in cases of changes to this scheme.

understanding, removing barriers for disabled people who want to work, and ensuring that disabled candidates can fulfil their potential.

There are three levels to the Disability Confident scheme. Level one is 'Disability Confident Committed'. At this level, employers agree to the Disability Confident commitments and identify at least one activity they will do to make a difference for disabled people. At level two – 'Disability Confident Employer' – employers must additionally complete a self-assessment and confirm that they are employing disabled people. At the final level – 'Disability Confident Leader' – employers must act as a disability champion within their local communities. Their self-assessment must be independently validated, and they must write a short statement saying what they have done or will to do be a Disability Confident Leader.

Disability Confident is a great scheme, and it's worth looking out for their logo on a company's website when you're deciding where you want to apply for a job. It can help to give you an idea of how committed employers are to advancing disability equity and is a sign that they guarantee an interview for disabled candidates who meet the essential job criteria.

Business Disability Forum

The Business Disability Forum (BDF) is the leading business membership organisation for disability inclusion in the UK. They work with business, government, and disabled employees to remove barriers to inclusion and improve their experiences of employment

182

and the workplace. BDF work with over 600 members, who employ around 20% of the UK workforce and an estimated 8 million people across the globe. They encourage businesses to become disability-aware and help to raise the voices of disabled employees to influence disability employment policy. In so doing, BDF create change in business practices, products, services, and policies to both benefit business and to improve the experiences of disabled employees.

The Business Disability Forum offers a great deal in its membership, including access to an international community of businesses. Members can further access specialist advice and opportunities through events, webinars, research, and collaborative networks. There are plenty of practical resources available on their extensive Knowledge Hub, as well as opportunities to participate in ongoing research. Joining the BDF demonstrates a business' commitment to disability equity and to becoming disability aware. It is a good idea to look out for the BDF logo on the websites of businesses that you're interested in working with, as it is evidence of their dedication to disability inclusion. Once you are part of a company that's a member of BDF, you'll get access to advice and support as a disabled employee of a member organisation.

What if you're disabled and can't work?

Whilst many disabled people can and do work, employment is by no means the best option for *all* disabled people. Some cannot work, or are retired on health grounds, and there should be no negative judgement about this. Each person must decide what is the best option for them. Even if you are unemployed, there are so many other ways to engage in your community, such as casual or voluntary work; these options may even be more flexible or accessible for you, working around your disability and access needs. It might be worth checking on casual work sites like Upwork to see if anything catches your eye or looking out for charities and voluntary organisations in your area.

If you are unable to work, there is still financial support available to you in the UK in the form of welfare benefits. These can help you to get some income to support yourself and contribute towards your disability-related needs. Unfortunately, disability can come with a hefty price tag. Research conducted by disability charity Scope in 2024 shows that, on average, disabled households need a staggering £1,010 per month more to have the same quality of living as non-disabled households.[19] Although benefits cannot cover the entirety of these costs, they can still help to offset them. Let's look at the main option for disability-related benefits in the UK, which is currently Personal Independence Payment (PIP).

---

[19] Scope. (2025) Disability Price Tag 2025 [Online]. Available at https://www.scope.org.uk/campaigns/disability-price-tag (Accessed 8 August 2025).

Personal Independence Payment (PIP)[20]

Personal Independence Payment, or PIP, can help with the extra costs associated with a disability if you have a long-term condition which causes you difficulty doing certain everyday tasks or getting around. You do not have to be unemployed to receive PIP; you can currently get it if you are working, if you are a student in Higher Education, if you have savings, or if you are on most other benefits. In early 2025, the Labour government proposed some changes to PIP, but – following resistance from disabled people, DPOs, and several MPs – these plans are now on hold pending the outcome of the Timms Review in autumn 2026.[21] However, let's briefly look at how the PIP system currently works.[22]

There are two components of Personal Independence Payment: a daily living component and a mobility component. You can receive either one or both parts at either a standard or an enhanced rate; how much you get will depend on how difficult you find certain tasks. You might receive the daily living component if you need help with

---

[20] Please note that all information was correct at time of publication [31 October 2025]. Please always check Government websites for the most up-to-date information in cases of changes to this scheme.

[21] Community Care. (1 July 2025) Government shelves personal independence payment cut in last-ditch concession to win welfare vote [Online]. Available at https://www.communitycare.co.uk/2025/07/01/government-shelves-personal-independence-payment-cut-in-last-ditch-concession-to-win-welfare-vote/ (Accessed 8 August 2025).

[22] Please note that all information was correct at time of publication [31 October 2025]. Please always check Government websites for the most up-to-date information in cases of changes to this scheme.

things like preparing food, toileting, washing and bathing, getting (un)dressed, managing money and socialising. You might get the mobility part if you have difficulty working out and following a route or if you find it hard to physically move around and leave your home. At present, each task is assessed on four key criteria:

- Whether you can do it safely.

- How long it takes you.

- How often your condition affects this activity.

- Whether you need help to do it, for instance, from another person, an aid, or a piece of adaptive equipment.

At present, you can apply for PIP if you are 16 or over, have a long-term physical disability or mental health condition, have difficulty doing any of the tasks outlined above, and you expect the difficulties to last for at least 12 months. Receiving PIP might qualify you for other kinds of support too. For example, if you get the mobility part of PIP, you might be eligible for a blue badge, vehicle tax discount or exemption, or a Motability scheme vehicle – more on this in chapter nine. If you receive the daily living component of PIP, you could apply for a Disabled Person's Railcard, or you might be able to get a discount on Council Tax and local bus travel. If someone helps to care for you, then they may be able to get Carer's Allowance or Carer's Credit.

Personal Independence Payment is a good scheme and a lifeline for many disabled people in the UK, whether they work or not. However, many disabled people find it a difficult process to go

186

through, and many do not receive the support they need on an initial application. Thankfully, there are plenty of organisations which can offer support in appealing the decision, including Citizens Advice, Scope, or PIP Help CIC. Whilst the application process can take a while, and it can be difficult to receive support, it is worth persevering to access the support that you need. If you need any help filling out your PIP application, you could ask someone in your support circle to help you. Citizens Advice or PIP Help CIC can sometimes offer support with the application process too, if you need it.

Some final thoughts...

Employment and education both offer brilliant avenues to develop your skills, do something that you feel is meaningful, and to earn financial security for yourself and your family. They can also contribute to other goals you may have, such as travelling or buying a house. But education and employment are not the right choice for everyone. You might not work in a traditional manner – or you might not work at all – due to your disability, and that is perfectly fine. We must each make the best choice for our body and mind, and only we can know what that is, despite what other people may say.

If you choose to pursue education or employment, there is a range of support out there to help you to navigate your time at university or in the workplace. This may be agreeing reasonable adjustments with your institution or employer or choosing to pursue additional support through either Disabled Students' Allowances or Access to Work. Receiving the right kind of support for you can be revolutionary and, for some, it might be the deciding factor as to whether you can remain in education or employment altogether. With the range of support out there in education and employment for disabled students and colleagues, never let anyone or anything stand in the way of you pursuing the course or job of your dreams! Remember, the world is your oyster!

What I learned:

- Know your rights as a disabled person in education or employment and never be afraid to advocate for yourself.

- You are entitled to reasonable adjustments in education and employment. Work with your institution or employer to get these put in place – it's about giving you an equitable chance to thrive and succeed in comparison to non-disabled people.

- It pays – quite literally – to do your research into grants and charitable awards to help get you the equipment that you need to succeed in education or employment. There is support out there, you just may need to do some investigation.

- Disclosing your disability to an education provider or employer is a very personal decision. There is no right or wrong answer, only the answer that feels the best for *you*.

- You may unfortunately face discrimination in education and employment, and this can have an immense impact on your confidence and self-esteem. Remember that discrimination often comes from a place of ignorance, and that there are support systems out there to help you when you encounter these difficulties.

- Not all disabled people can work or participate in education, and that is perfectly ok. We all must do what is best for us and our disabilities. If you cannot work, there is support out there in the form of PIP and UC. Don't hesitate to reach out for the support you need.

Reflection Time

1. If you're in further or higher education, what reasonable adjustments do you think would help you to thrive and succeed at your studies?

2. If you're in further or higher education, what steps will you take to put support in place for your disability? You might want to include connecting with your institution's disabled students' service, applying for DSAs and charity grants, or joining the disabled students' society.

3. If you're in employing or applying for jobs, when would you feel most comfortable disclosing your disability to an employer, and why?

4. If you're in work, what reasonable adjustments do you think would support you in your job? What steps will you take to put these

in place? You might want to think about talking to your line manager or HR.

5. If you're in work, is there any additional support you need? You might want to think about applying for Access to Work or getting support from the BDF.

6. If you're in work or study, are there any welfare benefits that you can apply for to help you with disability-related costs?

Chapter 7
You Gotta Fight for Your Rights!

Advocacy, ableism, and medical gaslighting

Whilst many disabled advocates are campaigning to improve things for us all, the world we currently live in is still not an equitable place for disabled people. Although we have come far in the last half-century thanks to the disability rights movement, there is still much farther to go in achieving disability equity. Even in today's political climate, some of the already hard-won freedoms that we enjoy are under threat of being repealed. Recently, section 504 of the Rehabilitation Act of 1973 – a US federal law that prohibits discrimination against people with disabilities – has come under fire from the American administration. In the UK, following the Labour government's green paper, over 1 million disabled people are expected to lose the financial support of their disability benefits completely, forcing them into poverty. For those disabled people who must regularly interact with the medical establishment, medical gaslighting is a common experience, especially for those with disabilities or chronic illnesses which are still poorly understood in mainstream medicine.

Facing inequality, (internalised) ableism, and medical gaslighting is sadly part of the disabled experience today, and one which still affects women and young disabled people

191

disproportionately. This is why it is so important to know and understand your rights, and to be able to advocate for yourself. This chapter will consider current disabled rights in the UK, how to advocate for yourself, how to deal with (internalised) ableism, and how to address medical gaslighting. I hope to support you in starting to build the skills which will stand you in good stead and help you to keep advancing disability equity in our society.

Your rights – the Equality Act 2010[23]

The Equality Act 2010 is a key piece of equality legislation in the UK. It covers people who have a disability, which it defines as someone with a physical or mental impairment that substantially and in the long-term limits their ability to undertake daily activities.[24] If you have a disability according to this definition, you can use the Equality Act 2010 to protect yourself against discrimination in work, education, or in services provided to you by businesses, organisations, and government departments in the UK. The Equality Act 2010 requires employers, education providers, and businesses to make reasonable adjustments to ensure that disabled people are included, that venues and services are accessible, and that disabled

---

[23] Please note that all information was correct at time of publication [31 October 2025]. Please always check Government websites for the most up-to-date information in cases of changes to laws.

[24] UK Government, (2010) Definition of disability under the Equality Act 2010 [Online]. Available at https://www.gov.uk/definition-of-disability-under-equality-act-2010 (Accessed 8 August 2025).

people have equitable access compared to their non-disabled counterparts.

The Equality Act 2010 further protects you from various kinds of discrimination due to your disability. This can include direct discrimination, such as where you are treated less favourably than others due to your disability. It similarly protects against indirect discrimination, such as if an employer or education provider has rules which put you at an unfair disadvantage as a disabled person. The Equality Act 2010 also protects you if you are being harassed or victimised due to your disability. These protections from discrimination apply in many situations, including buying or renting property, in education and employment, for transport, or for goods and services. If you think that you have been treated unfairly or discriminated against, you can complain directly to the person or organisation concerned, use someone like a union representative to help you to settle the matter, or make a claim in court or at a tribunal. Disability Rights UK's *Equality Advisory Support Service (EASS)* can assist you in such cases, as well as advising about reasonable adjustments to help you. You can either phone them, use their online contact form, or access their webcam portal for BSL users.

Stigma, ableism, and disability hate crimes

Ableism, or disablism, are both ways of describing the discrimination that disabled people experience. Ableism is the more frequently used term and refers to discrimination in favour of non-

193

disabled people. In an ableist society, then, it is assumed that the 'normal' way to live is as a non-disabled person. This attitude assumes that the physical, sensory, mental, or cognitive differences that people with disabilities experience are deficits; this is itself rooted in the medical model of disability whereby these perceived 'deficits' need to be fixed in some way. Ableism is manifest in the physical and attitudinal barriers that disabled people still face every day in our society, which is rarely built with them in mind. Some commonplace examples of ableism might include making assumptions, using derogatory language, asking intrusive questions, excluding disabled people, or using accessible facilities designed for disabled people when you don't need them. We shall look at how to combat ableism in greater depth in the self-advocacy section later in this chapter.

Disability discrimination arises when you're treated differently because of your disability. This might include being passed over for a job or being denied entry to a building, or if your employer, school, or university fail to make reasonable adjustments for you. Disability stigma comprises the negative attitudes and beliefs about disabled people which can lead to discrimination and exclusion. Disability stigmas can present in many ways, such as stereotyping, social avoidance, or even hate crimes and violence. There are so many stereotypes about disability which are simply not true. Some people assume, for instance, that everyone with a disability is a benefit scrounger, when most disabled people do not have access to benefits and, for those that do, the fraud rate for PIP applications fell to 0% in 2023-24.[25] Stigma and stereotypes can have a profound impact on disabled people's lives because they are so pervasive; they can affect our quality of life and wellbeing, as well as our access to education, employment, and healthcare.

If you experience or witness ableism or disability discrimination, there are several avenues to report it and make sure that you do not face this alone. If you experience discrimination at work, talk to your line manager as your first port of call, as they may be able to help you to resolve the situation. If this doesn't help, you could report the incident to HR as soon as possible – your employer should then take this very seriously. If a business or service provider discriminates against you due to your disability, try to raise your concern as quickly as possible with a member of staff or the manager. You can then follow-up the incident in writing to explain what happened and to ask for an update on how the business will deal with this in future. You could also ask for the complaints procedure to pick this up if you would like to make a formal complaint. If you experience disability discrimination in Higher Education, speak with your personal tutor to receive pastoral support

---

[25] UK Government. (16 May 2024) Fraud and error in the benefit system, Financial Year Ending (FYE) 2024 [Online]. Available at https://www.gov.uk/government/statistics/fraud-and-error-in-the-benefit-system-financial-year-2023-to-2024-estimates/fraud-and-error-in-the-benefit-system-financial-year-ending-fye-2024#personal-independence-payment-overpayments-and-underpayments (Accessed 8 August 2025).

and follow your university or college's formal procedure for reporting such incidents.

One extreme form of disability discrimination is hate crime. A disability hate crime happens when someone targets a person because they are disabled, and can take many forms, including physical attacks, assault on assistance animals, threat of attack such as threatening letters or texts, harassment, or bullying and abuse online, at school, or in the workplace. The police have a duty to investigate hate crimes and will decide whether an incident has occurred. Telling the police about hate crimes will help them to keep you safe, and it may protect other disabled people from a similar fate too. You can report a hate crime as the victim, as a witness, or on behalf of a friend or family member. Before you make a report, you might want to think of all the information you will need, as it can be upsetting to talk about such incidents. If the incident is affecting your mental health, you can ask for support from the police, Victim Support, or disability charities such as Scope. If you do not wish to talk to the police directly, you can report a hate crime anonymously through a third-party reporting centre run by local agencies, such as Citizens Advice.

Internalised ableism

As well as ableism, you may have heard people in the disability community or social media influencers talking about 'internalised ableism'. Internalised ableism refers to the impact that living in an

196

ableist society and constantly being on the receiving end of ableism can have upon us. Sometimes, for instance, disabled people might have low self-esteem or a sense of shame about their disability due to internalised ableism. This is essentially when a disabled person has continuous exposure to negative social attitudes and a lack of adequate support for their needs, and so they absorb these ableist views, especially the belief that disability is a source of shame. As societal awareness of disability rights and equity has grown in recent decades, there has been an increasing recognition of internalised ableism as a significant barrier to the wellbeing and self-esteem of disabled people. Internalised oppression – including internalised ableism – can lead to the normalisation of practices, policies, or behaviours which systematically exclude and marginalise certain groups in society, such as disabled people. This deeply affects how they see themselves and others within their group.

So, what can we do to combat our own internalised ableism? Remember that you have spent a long time – potentially even your whole life – being conditioned in an ableist society, and so dismantling your own *internalised* ableism is a task that will take time and effort. Being in a place to resist internalised ableism further depends on whether you have access to safer spaces where disabled people feel welcome and supported. Such spaces are essential to create a sense of solidarity, belonging, and empowerment. You might find these kinds of spaces in support groups for your disability or for disabled people in general. Alternatively, you might want to reach out to the vast disability community online or on social media. The support of your (chosen) family and friends also plays a pivotal role in helping you to dismantle your internalised ableism. They can again create a supportive environment in which you can more safely challenge ableist ideas and explore alternatives.

Another thing which might help with internalised ableism is to learn about the social model of disability, rather than the medical model. This enables you to see disability not as the result of a physical or mental 'flaw' or 'deficit', but instead as arising from society's ableist attitudes and its lack of support for disabled people – factors that *can* be changed; you can find out more about the social model of disability in chapter two.

Another way to battle internalised ableism is to practice self-love, to unlearn the beliefs that society has taught you about having a disability, and to believe unwaveringly in your own self-worth. Although society has trained us to believe that our worth is dependent on having a non-disabled body or mind, being disabled does *not* make you any less worthy of love and happiness. We have inherent worth that is found by looking inside each person. To help you unlearn such attitudes and believe in your inherent worth, surround yourself by others in the disability community. After all, if you wouldn't judge them for their differences or believe them to be unworthy of love and happiness, why would you continue to judge yourself in this manner? When you experience these moments of internalised ableism, recognise them in your mind, challenge them, and call them out. But be kind and gentle with yourself too, as it will take time and effort to unlearn all of this. Try not to be too hard on yourself if you do get internalised ableist thoughts, as it is just how society has conditioned us to think. Instead, view it as an opportunity to challenge this type of internalised ableism and to grow as a person capable of challenging these views.

Medical Gaslighting

Medical gaslighting is another thing that disabled people ought to be aware of, especially if your disability or condition mean that you need regular medical appointments or treatment. Medical gaslighting is when a medical professional dismisses a patient's physical symptoms or attributes them to something else, such as a psychological condition. It is more likely to happen to women, disabled people, and people from minoritised ethnic groups. There are several reasons why medical gaslighting may occur. The healthcare provider may have poor communication skills, have limited time to speak with the patient, or may not be medically knowledgeable enough to know what to do, especially if you have a rare disease or are a medically complex case. Medical gaslighting could stem from having a disability or condition that still isn't well understood, such as ME/ CFS or Long COVID.

You might have experienced medical gaslighting if a healthcare provider doesn't listen to you or interrupts you, if they diminish your symptoms, if they blame your symptoms on anxiety or on your gender, ethnicity, weight or lifestyle habits, or if they rush you through the appointment. Most doctors do not intentionally gaslight patients, but they often get so little time with each person that it makes it difficult to share detailed information and answer questions fully.

Women are unfortunately more likely than men to have their symptoms attributed to a mental health condition. One study has indicated that women with pain were less likely than men with the same issues to receive pain medication, and even where they received it, they had to wait much longer than their male counterparts.[26] Research also shows that health institutes have generally overfunded research on diseases that affect men and underfunded research on health issues which mainly affect women.[27] As a result, medical professionals are less knowledgeable about women's health issues, needs, and treatments. The same applies to race, as Black, Asian, and Latino/a/x people are more

---

[26] King's College London. (4 September 2024) Study finds women less likely to be prescribed pain relief than men [Online]. Available at https://www.kcl.ac.uk/news/study-finds-women-less-likely-to-be-prescribed-pain-relief-than-men#:~:text=In%20a%20study%20of%20thousands,in%20emergency%20departments%20for%20longer. (Accessed 8 August 2025).

[27] Jamie White & Janine Clayton. (13 May 2022) The gender health innovation gap: A perspective from the NIH office of research on women's health [Online]. Available at https://www.sciencedirect.com/science/article/pii/S2666634022001763#:~:text=Despite%20ongoing%20efforts%2C%20women's%20health,6 (Accessed 8 August 2025).

likely to have their stroke symptoms misdiagnosed than their white counterparts.[28]

Medical gaslighting can affect people in both physically and emotionally damaging ways. If patients are not believed, they may spend a long time trying to find a doctor who will listen and accurately diagnose their condition. This may result in excessive (and possibly very expensive) tests, potential misdiagnosis, and physical pain from the failure to address a medical condition with appropriate care. The emotional distress associated with medical gaslighting can have long-lasting psychological effects, leading patients to develop anxiety, depression, and potentially PTSD.

Medical gaslighting ultimately leads to worse medical outcomes for patients. There is an urgent need to reform our healthcare systems, and to allow doctors to spend adequate time with each patient to listen to their concerns, and for them to have the required resources to make an accurate diagnosis.

Whilst reforming our entire healthcare system will take time and government involvement, there is plenty that disabled people can do to tackle medical gaslighting when they encounter it. Perhaps most important – but most difficult of all – is to find a doctor that you

---

[28] Ellis Charles & Leonard Egede. (2008) Ethnic disparities in stroke recognition in individuals with prior stroke [Online]. Available at https://pmc.ncbi.nlm.nih.gov/articles/PMC2430648/#:~:text=Racial/ethnic%20d ifferences%20in%20recognition%20of%20signs%20of%20stroke,%25)%20resp ondents%20(Table%202). (Accessed 8 August 2025).

trust. If you ever feel that a doctor is dismissing your symptoms, talking down to you, or not listening to you, you are perfectly within your rights to search around for someone who listens to you, answers your questions, and takes your concerns seriously. If you do have a difficult doctor, you could bring a trusted friend or family member with you to appointments for support. This way, you will have someone there who can back you up if your doctor begins to question your symptoms. Your friend or family member may remember details or think of questions that might not have occurred to you as well.

Another tactic to defend against medical gaslighting is to go into the appointment as prepared as possible. You could bring a journal to track the symptoms you've been having, or a list of questions you want to ask. It can help to write your symptoms and questions down, either on paper or in the note's app on your phone to ensure that all your concerns are being addressed. If possible, it might help to track your symptoms over time to give your doctor more data, especially if your condition fluctuates. You might want to take more notes during your appointment too, so that you can refer to what was said and agreed later. Finally, if you're not happy with the outcome from your doctor, you can always ask for a second opinion. This might be helpful if you feel that a doctor from a different speciality might be able to better understand and address your concerns.

Experiencing medical gaslighting can be an immensely hard and, at times, harrowing experience, especially on top of living with a disability, neurodiverse, or chronic health condition. It can make you question your symptoms, whether they are really 'all in your head', as well as doubt whether there is anything actually 'wrong' with you. In these instances, it's important to remember that *you* know your body best and if you sense that something is off, you're most likely to be right. Try to analyse your interactions with medical professionals and identify medical gaslighting when it occurs. If you feel like you are being gaslit by a medical professional, remember that you can always search for another doctor and a second opinion. You deserve a doctor who will listen to you, take your concerns seriously, and act in your best interests to support your health. A key part in tackling medical gaslighting is therefore to advocate for yourself and your needs. But what exactly is self-advocacy, and why is it important for disabled individuals?

Self-Advocacy

Self-advocacy is the ability to speak up for yourself and to request that your needs are met, because *you* know what is in *your* best interests. It's important to speak up for what you need and want so that you can get the best support and make the most out of your life. Self-advocacy can help you to make choices, take responsibility, and exercise your rights. As disabled people, learning to be a self-advocate is of the utmost importance. Unfortunately, there are likely to be many occasions in your life that call on you to advocate for yourself and your access needs, whether that's in education, employment, or going about your daily life.

There are many key qualities that a successful self-advocate embodies. If you wish to advocate for yourself, you will first need to know what it is that you want to obtain or achieve. Once this is settled, you will need to be confident enough to ask for what you want and to make decisions for yourself. It can help if you understand your own strengths and weaknesses as a self-advocate.

Sometimes, though, we can find it hard to advocate for ourselves in certain situations for a variety of reasons. You might find it difficult to assert yourself to those who are in positions of power over you like a line manager or a university tutor. You might worry about how you communicate or find it hard to get your point across and your voice heard. You might be unused to speaking out and having people listen to you, or you may be concerned what will happen if you speak out – for instance, will people at work see you as a troublemaker if you speak up and assert your needs?

These are all valid concerns that could stand in the way of your journey to becoming a successful self-advocate. However, there are various things that you can do to help build your confidence to advocate for yourself. Firstly, it can help to have a plan. By thinking about *what* you want and *how* you want to achieve this, the actions that you will need to take as a self-advocate will become clearer. You might want to plan out who you need to speak with and the best way to do this, for example, when and where should you meet, and what will you say to them? If you are nervous, it can help to have a script or prompt for the points you want to cover. You may want to ask a friend or family member to rehearse the interaction with you ahead of time and give you some feedback on how you can improve.

When it comes to advocating for yourself, it can help to understand your rights as a disabled person in the UK, such as under the Equality Act 2010. Effective communication is another key quality of a successful self-advocate. You could practice active listening, which entails paying close attention to the speaker, understanding what they're saying, and responding appropriately. You might wish to practice expressing yourself clearly and concisely, and think about *how* you want to communicate, whether that be face-to-face, on the telephone, or via video chat. If you are feeling anxious or need someone to help keep you on track, you could request a chaperone to join you in the meeting and offer some support. Whilst it is important to be confident and believe in what you are saying, it is helpful to remain open to feedback too, as successful communication is a two-way process. You could also agree to keep a shared written record of what is said and agreed in the meeting, to ensure that everyone remains accountable for their actions.

Having considered how to be a successful self-advocate, it's time to look at these skills in practice, especially when it comes to addressing everyday instances of ableism. This might include things like videos not having captions or BSL interpretation, ramps not being available for wheelchair users to traverse steps, stereotyping disabled people as either tragic victims or sources of inspiration porn, or asking a disabled person what is 'wrong' with them. Everyday ableism can comprise ableist language, including many phrases that most people say unthinkingly, such as saying 'blind as a bat', 'deaf as a post', or calling something 'lame' or 'crazy'; all are ableist slurs.

By advocating for ourselves, though, disabled people can combat such waves of everyday ableism. Self-advocates can ask for what they need to participate in certain activities, encourage others to listen to disabled voices, or promote inclusive practice in everything that they do. At the same time, it's important to remember that disability is not homogenous and is intersectional with other marginalised groups and protected characteristics, and so our activism needs to be intersectional too. Self-advocates might seek out views from diverse members of the disabled community and use their privilege to amplify the voices of other minoritised communities. They might further promote the social model of disability and actively encourage disability equity wherever they can. If we self-advocate together, we can achieve a lot of change in this world.

Whilst cultivating the skills of a successful self-advocate is crucial for many disabled people, this role does not come without its own challenges. Sometimes, it can feel like the onus is entirely on you as a disabled person to advocate for your needs and to promote disability equity within your spheres of influence. This role can feel incredibly draining, especially if you are self-advocating for your needs without the support of the wider disability community, which can be a source of strength. This is why allies are so crucial to efforts to advance disability equity too. Although 20% of the UK population is disabled, 1 in 3 disabled people still feel that there is a lot of prejudice towards them.[29] Such stigma and prejudice will not simply disappear on its own, or with the efforts of disabled self-advocates. We need the wider support of disabled allies to turn the tide of prejudice. But what is an ally, and how can you become one for disabled people?

How to be an ally to disabled people

In our society, disabled people should not have to be the ones to constantly advocate for themselves and their needs. Indeed, disability is the only minoritised group that *anyone* can join at *any time*, and that most people are likely to join if they grow to be old enough. Disability equity should be a shared concern *for us all*, then, and we have a collective responsibility to be good allies to disabled

---

[29] Scope. (22 May 2018) Disabled people still face negative attitudes [Online]. Available at https://www.scope.org.uk/news-and-stories/disabled-people-still-face-negative-attitudes#:~:text=What%20is%20the%20Perception%20Gap,calling%20the%20disability%20perception%20gap. (Accessed 8 August 2025).

people. But what is an ally? Allies play an important role in changing attitudes and removing barriers for the marginalised groups they support by using their privilege to effect change. Allies listen carefully to disabled people, speak out against injustice, and take action to make the world a more inclusive, accessible, and equitable place for disabled people to live in. Allies should not speak on behalf of disabled people, though, but should instead seek to amplify their voices.

Allyship is one way of taking responsibility for embedding change and being inclusive within our society. Being a disability ally does not necessarily mean that you are an expert on all disability-related matters. It instead means that you are actively listening to disabled people, showing your support, and educating others about disability and accessibility issues. There are several ways to be a good ally to disabled people, including:

- **Treating disabled people equitably** with the way you treat everyone else.

- **Educate yourself.** Read up on the privilege you have as a non-disabled person or learn more about disability and accessibility. You could read books by disabled authors or follow disabled influencers on your favourite social media platform. You might want to learn about different kinds of disability too, or the social and medical models of disability – chapter two has more information on this.

- **Listen to disabled people and amplify their voices.** Disabled people often struggle to get their voices heard due to the prejudice and discrimination which persist in our society. But we have a saying in disability advocacy, 'nothing about us without us'. It is an essential part of being an ally to talk to disabled people, listen to what we have to say, and use your privilege to amplify our voices.

- **Do not assume.** Many disabilities are less apparent than others, meaning that – whilst they can impact on a person's daily life tremendously – you cannot tell just by looking at that person what challenges they are facing. Do not assume whether someone is disabled or not just by looking at them; you can't judge a book by its cover when it comes to disabilities.

- **Speak out and support.** If you see prejudice, stigma, or discrimination, speak up. Good allies report or challenge this kind of behaviour wherever they see it. You might act in a variety of different ways, but it's always a good idea to check in with the disabled person who has been affected and ask them what kind of support they would like to receive in the situation.

- **Be open to feedback.** As an ally, you will never get everything right all the time, as you are not living as a disabled person. Therefore, be willing to adjust your actions or attitudes based on what you learn, or if a disabled person points out something that you could improve on. At the end of the day, it will make you an even better ally!

- **Amplify disabled creators' content.** There are lots of disabled people who use their social media platforms to educate others, change perceptions, and raise awareness around disability equity. Repost or boost their content, as it lifts disabled creators' voices and shows your support for their content. Plus, you're actively educating yourself and others by sharing this kind of content!

- **Think about accessibility in everything you do.** As a disabled ally, thinking about accessibility should be an integral part of your life. Whether you directly benefit from accessibility or not, it should always be on your radar, and you should educate others where you can.

These are only a few ways to be a good ally to disabled people. Allies play a very important role in promoting disability equity and in creating a more inclusive and accessible world. Never underestimate the impact you can have as an ally!

Nevertheless, being an ally can bring its own challenges and be difficult at times. There are several factors that might prevent allies from acting and speaking up in certain situations. It is important to identify and acknowledge these factors, as this is the first step in tackling them. Some reasons which prevent allies from being effective include:

- **Fear.** Fear can be a considerable barrier, as allies might worry about doing or saying the 'wrong thing' and unintentionally causing more harm than good. This can lead to allies becoming frozen in inactivity. It's crucial to recognise that making mistakes is a natural part of life and of the learning process. Alternatively, you could use your fear to motivate you to better educate yourself and to build your knowledge, so that you do not experience this fear again.

- **Social pressure.** Social pressure can make it hard to be an ally, especially if allies fear ostracism for speaking out on issues. This kind of social pressure can again lead to inaction. Whilst speaking out or acting on behalf of disabled people might be uncomfortable, change cannot happen without it. It might first be easier to find communities or groups who align with your values and views, so that you can practice speaking out as part of a group who share your opinions before moving on to potentially tougher crowds.

- **Burn out.** Allyship and advocacy can be physically and emotionally tiring, and so some allies struggle with fatigue, burnout, or loss of momentum over time. To avoid burn-out, prioritise your own self-care routines and rest, as well as connecting with the disabled community or other allies who can offer empathy and support. Allyship is a marathon, not a sprint, and so pacing yourself well is important to keep momentum going; you can find out more about how to look after your wellbeing in chapter eight. Remember too that you do not have to undergo your allyship journey alone – find others in the same boat who can help to support you!

- **Lack of knowledge.** If you are new to allyship or just starting out on your allyship journey, you may not know where to start or how best to support the disabled community, as you are yet to build your knowledge base of the key issues affecting disabled people in our society today. There is an easy fix to this one – commit to educating yourself on these issues by reading books, listening to podcasts, looking at resources, or following disabled influencers and creators on social media. You might want to seek out opportunities to engage with members of the disabled community through group meetups or chat boards for support groups.

- **Privilege.** Allies may struggle to recognise their own privilege or may feel uncomfortable about the privilege that they hold given that it contributes to the marginalisation and discrimination of others. This can prevent allies from really engaging with members of the community they seek to support and understanding their lived experiences. Allies who experience this could commit to dismantling their privilege through self-reflection and education. Whilst this may be an uncomfortable experience at first, it can help you to actively listen to and learn from marginalised voices and deeply understand the community that you want to support. You could then seek out opportunities to use your privilege to amplify the voices of the disabled community, such as sharing the work of disabled activists, creators, and influencers.

Although being an ally might not be easy at times, it's an immensely rewarding and worthwhile role to undertake to support the disabled community, or another marginalised group. Being an ally can also be tremendous fun – it can expand your horizons and encourage you to make connections and socialise with a group or community that you might otherwise have overlooked. If you want to be a good ally to disabled people, educate yourself, listen carefully to them, and use your privilege to amplify their voices. With the help of allies, we can create long-lasting change more quickly and more effectively than if disabled people had to continually self-advocate on their own!

Some final thoughts...

Unfortunately, we do not live in a perfect or equitable world for disabled people, which means that there are still so many things to fight and self-advocate for. Ours is a world in which internalised ableism and medical gaslighting persist, damaging disabled people's confidence and self-esteem. Those who are meant to help and support us, such as medical professionals, can sometimes do more harm than good. But there is hope in the growth of allies and in the disabled community increasingly self-advocating for their needs. Together, we have a collective responsibility to improve life for disabled people, as you never know when *you* or someone you love might join this minoritised and marginalised group. By learning to be a good self-advocate or a good ally, you will be going a long way to supporting disabled people and fighting for disability equity in this sometimes messed up, at other times wonderful world.

What I learned:

- Learn your rights as a disabled person and don't be afraid to advocate for yourself – you are worthy of support, respect, and being treated with dignity.

- Unfortunately, we live in a world that can be ableist and inaccessible, and one in which stigma and discrimination persist. Remember that discrimination often arises out of ignorance, and that is it no reflection upon you as a disabled person. Find support where you can.

- A lot of disabled people struggle with internalised ableism, even though we rarely talk about it, so remember that you are not alone. Try to dismantle these beliefs if you can and surround yourself with the love and support of your loved ones and the disability community to lift you up.

- Medical gaslighting is sadly common and is more likely to occur for women. But remember that doctors do not always know everything and that *you* know *your* body the best. If you experience medical gaslighting, know that you can always ask for a second opinion and challenge your doctor, and seek support from a loved one who can help to advocate for you.

- Self-advocacy is important but so are allies who can advocate alongside us.

- If you want to be a better ally to disabled people, educate yourself about disability, think about accessibility in everything that you do, listen to disabled people and amplify their voices, and remain open to feedback from the disability community.

Reflection Time:

1. Do you experience any internalised ableism? How does it make you feel? Can you think of any ways you could challenge these thoughts?

2. Have you ever faced any medical gaslighting? How did it feel, and how did you deal with it? If you were ever in that situation again, would you react differently or is there anything you would change?

3. How will you self-advocate for yourself as a disabled person going forwards? What qualities of a successful self-advocate do you already have, and which might you need to cultivate?

4. If you're reading this book as an ally, what steps will you take to become a (better) ally? Is there anything that holds you back as an ally, and how can you address this?

Chapter 8
Finding Your Zen

Pacing, mental health, and wellbeing

As you may have gathered by now, when you're disabled, you may encounter additional challenges with your physical or mental health, which non-disabled people do not have to face. Whether it's accessing support at work, fighting for accessibility, or dealing with discrimination, having a disability can bring its fair share of additional challenges that you just have to roll with. As well as looking after your wellbeing, if you live with an energy-limiting condition like ME/ CFS or Long Covid – or if fatigue is part of your disability – you may also need to learn how to pace your energy carefully to achieve all the things you want. This might be the case if you experience a lot of chronic pain, too. This chapter will look at what pacing is and how to implement it, as well as my top tips for managing your mental health and wellbeing with a disability or dealing with chronic pain. Although I'm by no means an expert in mental health, I'm here to share the things that have helped me countless times, in the hope that they might ease things for you too. So, let's start with pacing.

Pacing – what on earth is it and how do I do it successfully?

If you have a chronic illness – or especially an energy-limiting condition – odds are that you've heard the word 'pacing' more than a few times already. So, what on earth is it and, more importantly, how do we pace our activity levels effectively? Many people experience fatigue as part of their disability. Fatigue is more than just 'feeling tired'; it is a debilitating condition that can leave you feeling drained or flu-like, where even resting does not significantly relieve this feeling. Fatigue is a symptom of many chronic illnesses and is a diagnostic criterion for certain conditions such as ME/ CFS and Long Covid. People with these kinds of conditions tend to find that symptoms such as pain, fatigue, brain fog, or muscle aches get worse after mental or physical exertion. This is called post-exertional malaise, or PEM. PEM can encompass fatigue, pain, cognitive dysfunction, and sleep disruption, among other symptoms. It is characterised by a delay in the onset of symptoms, which makes it hard to recognise when over-exertion is happening. This can lead to a debilitating cycle of relapsing and recovering, often referred to as the 'boom-and-bust cycle'.

Boom-and-bust is a pattern of activity where you do too much on a good day, which can lead to increased pain and fatigue in the following days, and with it the need to rest and reduce your activity to get back to your baseline. This cycle of over-exertion and relapse can make it harder to manage pain and fatigue over time. For instance, one morning you may wake up feeling great – you have so

217

much energy and you're in very little pain. So, you tackle a long list of tasks that you've been putting off. As this is your first good day in a while, you want to make the most of it, so you work hard and take very few breaks. But what happens on the day after? You wake up, your pain is through the roof, and you feel flu-like and absolutely drained. You don't think you can face getting out of bed, let alone eating breakfast or attempting the list of jobs you had to do today. So, you spend the day in bed, trying to distract yourself from the pain and worrying that you're entering a flare-up. For the next few days, you continue to feel drained, and your pain remains high – it seems you were right about that flare-up!

When you have a disability, it is natural to have better and worse days. But, as we've seen above, it is easy to become trapped in the boom-and-bust cycle. If these cycles persist, over time you will be able to do less, and your pain and fatigue will continue to get worse; you will have fewer good days, and it will take you longer to recover from your flare-ups. The trick is to manage your energy so that you can slowly build it up bit by bit to better cope with your pain and fatigue.

This is where pacing comes in. Pacing is essentially a strategy to manage your fatigue levels and minimise PEM by balancing rest and activity. It involves finding a comfortable range of energy expenditure for you which avoids over-exertion. The goal is to help people to feel better, to prevent symptoms from worsening, and to stabilise their condition. Pacing requires a few key steps:

- You need to learn to recognise your symptoms and any indicators that a flare-up is on the horizon.

- You need to plan activity in limited amounts and alternate it with periods of rest.

- You ought to avoid or limit activities which make your symptoms worse.

- You set realistic goals for when to gradually increase your energy expenditure.

By following these steps, pacing can help you to avoid boom-and-bust cycles, remain as active as possible, and limit the number and severity of your relapses. Although pacing sounds simple in principle, it can be hard to implement and perfect in practice. Many people find it frustrating at first, as finding that sweet spot between activity and rest can be immensely hard to achieve. Keeping a daily activity and symptom log can help to show you where you might be over-doing it so you can make changes. It might help for you to colour-code your log like a traffic light system and track your energy and symptom levels every 15-30 minutes or so. If you're feeling good and could carry on, it's green. If you're starting to feel unwell, it's amber. And if you're feeling awful and need to stop, it's red. This way, you'll be able to see when you hit amber so that you can learn to stop and rest before you get worse. Alternatively, you can break amber or red activities into smaller tasks, or intersperse them with green tasks, to manage your energy better. You might also want to be mindful of how many red or amber activities you plan within a day or week, as this could drain your energy or lead to a flare-up.

Even with good pacing management, it's important to remember that flare-ups and relapses are still going to happen, especially when you have a trigger. But pacing will help you to manage your symptoms for most of the time. It can help to build up your activity slowly with smaller amounts of energy and to prioritise tasks by focusing on the most important ones when you are feeling well. Remember to take plenty of breaks throughout the day too.

Pacing can become difficult when you have big tasks or events that you cannot avoid. Perhaps you're moving house or attending a friend's wedding as part of the bridal or groom party, a request which you could not refuse. You might be asking how you are meant to pace for these things? You may even feel anxious about whether your body can manage the event and its demands on you, and what effect this will have on you. On such occasions, the best course of action when it comes to pacing is:

- To make a sensible and realistic pacing plan and stick to it.

- Explain to others about your limitations and do not try to hide your problems.

- Find a suitable place where you can rest in quiet, and rest before you feel tired.

If you cannot get your pacing under control, it is worth speaking to your GP to ask for further support and to maybe get a referral to a service for chronic fatigue or energy-limiting conditions.

One of the most challenging days on which I had to pace my pain and fatigue levels was my wedding day. This was before I became a full-time wheelchair user, back when I could sometimes stand and walk for limited distances. I knew that this would be a big day, with many demands on me as the bride, and that I would not make it through unless I put a realistic pacing plan in place. We planned the ceremony for the afternoon, to give me plenty of time to rest and get ready in the morning at a leisurely pace. When selecting our venue, we chose one with a small secondary room that could be used exclusively by the bridal party, which gave me a little oasis to retreat to if I needed to rest or if things became too overwhelming. I had also chosen a long wedding dress with long sleeves, which meant I could conceal my joint braces, KT tape, and other aids which relieved my pain beneath my clothing, as well as my comfy shoes. By devising a suitable pacing plan and sticking to it, as well as finding a quiet space to rest in when required, we made our wedding day so much more manageable from a pacing point of view.

The Spoon Theory

Another way to think about pacing is through something called the Spoon Theory. This was developed by Christine Miserando, who has a chronic illness and who was trying to explain to her friend what it was like to live with this condition. The Spoon Theory is a metaphor to help others to understand how chronic conditions and disabilities limit a person's energy for daily tasks. Miserando explained it to her friend like this: she grabbed a bunch of nearby spoons and told her friend that each one represented a unit of energy that she could spend on tasks throughout the day. People who are not living with energy-limiting conditions or disabilities often wake up with an unlimited number of spoons, meaning they do not have to think about how they will budget their energy. But disabled people wake up with a limited number of spoons to spend on their daily tasks. The number of spoons that a person has may vary day to day depending on their symptoms, and the number of spoons that each task takes will vary between different people too. For instance, I might wake up with 12 spoons in a day. Getting breakfast might take 1 spoon, showering another 3, and brushing my teeth another 1. Before I'm ready to start my day, I've already used nearly half of my daily allowance. I may be able to 'borrow' spoons from the next day's allowance, but this means I'll start tomorrow in a deficit. Managing spoons means making important decisions about how and where we use our energies.

The Spoon Theory shows how people with chronic illnesses and disabilities often have limited energy compared to non-disabled people and how we must think carefully about how to budget this throughout the day. Spoon Theory can help disabled people to plan their day by deciding what's essential and what can be put off to another day, meaning that we're not always able to do everything we want. It can also help others to understand how their disability impacts their ability to work, socialise, or do other activities. The Spoon Theory has gathered something of a following amongst the disabled and chronically ill community. The hashtag #spoonies is growing on social media to unite and identify people who live with energy-limiting conditions, chronic illnesses, and disabilities.

Top tips for pacing

Pacing is something that you will get used to with time and better at with practice. However, here are some top tips that I've picked up along the way, and which have helped me to hone my pacing skills as someone with chronic fatigue:

- Don't try to use more energy than you think you have – you'll have to borrow from the next day's energy reserves, or it will push you into a boom-and-bust cycle.

- Do not try to 'push through' your symptoms – stop and rest instead.

- Learn to recognise the feeling of 'doing too much' and stop before you hit it.

- Aim to have some energy left by the end of the day.

- Try to stick to resting and relaxation during the day, rather than sleeping, as this could disturb your sleep cycle at night.

- Make use of aids and adaptations to help with mobility and everyday household tasks, as this will help you to pace more effectively.

- Try to make your plans for the day realistic, achievable, and sustainable.

- Once you have achieved a degree of stability, you can gradually increase the amount of physical and mental activity that you are doing.

- Give yourself permission to rest and relax and try not to feel any guilt – you are doing what's best for your body.

- It's helpful to plan ahead at the start of the day, once you know your energy budget.

- For more complicated tasks, think about how you can break these down into smaller, more manageable components and space rest breaks in between them.

- Learn to say no and ask for help. It is important to set and protect your boundaries, but it's crucial to recognise when you need help too, and to accept this.

Looking after your mental health with a disability

Over the past few decades, as a society we have become increasingly aware that we *all* have mental health and wellbeing that we need to look after. Mental health refers to our psychological and emotional state, whilst wellbeing refers to the state of being comfortable, happy, and healthy. With this growing awareness, support for those with mental health conditions has also grown. There is still a long way to go until we have an equitable society for people with mental health conditions, though, especially when it comes to accessing diagnosis and treatment in a timely manner or overcoming the stigma that is often associated with poor mental health.

Being disabled – whether it is a physical or mental health condition – presents unique challenges to our mental health and wellbeing. For me, for instance, living with severe chronic pain all the time has affected my mental health and wellbeing at times, throwing me into pits of depression and anxiety alongside pain flare-ups. The discrimination I've faced as a disabled woman has similarly had an impact on my mental health; when I was facing severe disability discrimination at one point in my life, my loved ones often said that I had become a shell of my former self who no longer genuinely smiled and who always looked sad and scared behind my eyes. This is a pretty good reflection of how broken I felt inside too at that time. These are challenges that non-disabled people may find hard to understand. But they are the reason why it's so important to look after your mental health and wellbeing when you are disabled, so that you can become resilient in the face of adversity.

The remainder of this chapter will contain some tips that I've learned along the way from pain and symptom management courses, through wellbeing services at work, and through my own knowledge, research, and trial and error. Some of these tips may seem obvious, or you may even question how they can help when you are facing serious mental health issues. Sometimes, it can feel like you're putting a sticking plaster over a shark bite. But implementing these tips has helped me to build the foundations for a balanced and calming life, and to face mental health dips head-on when they've occurred, instead of feeling completely at sea. My hope is that some of these tips will help you to manage the mental health and wellbeing challenges that come with disability even just a little bit more easily.

Sleep

Multiple research studies have shown that there is a close relationship between sleep and mental health.[30] Living with a mental health condition can affect how well you can sleep, and poor sleep

---

[30] Mental Health Foundation. (2020) Taking Sleep Seriously [Online]. Available at https://www.mentalhealth.org.uk/sites/default/files/2022-07/MHF-Taking-Sleep-Seriously-Publication-2020.pdf (Accessed 8 August 2025).

has a negative impact on your mental health, potentially leading to a vicious circle. Sleep is just as important when you live with a disability or chronic illness, but it can often be a problematic area for many disabled people. You might find it hard to fall and stay asleep or you might wake up earlier than you'd like; if this happens frequently, it's known as insomnia. Others in the disability community experience what they term 'painsomnia', an endless loop where poor sleep leads to increased pain, and high pain levels disrupt sleep. Due to insomnia or painsomnia, you might find it hard to wake up and get out of bed, or you may feel tired or sleepy during the day as you're not getting enough good-quality sleep at night. Alternatively, some disabled people experience the problem where they sleep too much, which is known as narcolepsy – a chronic condition that affects the brain's ability to control sleep-wake cycles. Some people may even have experiences that disturb their sleep, such as panic attacks, nightmares, or night terrors.

There are many other factors related to disability which can cause additional problems affecting our sleep. To name but a few, stresses, worries, and anxiety can disrupt our sleep by keeping us awake. There might be problems with where you sleep, such as not having a bed that is supportive enough or your room being too light or too hot or cold to facilitate good sleep. Starting or coming off different medications may result in side effects which impact on your sleep cycle too. There may be social factors that impact on how well you sleep; being a parent or carer, for instance, or working night shifts. Current or past trauma, as well as mental or physical health problems and neurodivergent conditions, can all affect how much and how well we sleep as well.

There are many ways in which our sleep cycles could be disrupted by physical or mental health conditions and disabilities. If you have sleep problems, this could make your mental health worse; those who do not sleep well are more likely to feel anxious or depressed and might even be affected by certain mental health conditions. If you cannot sleep, you may feel lonely and isolated if you do not have the energy to see the people you want, or if you feel like they don't understand what you're going through. Lack of sleep can cause you to be more affected by physical health problems too, including fatigue and chronic pain, leading you to feel that your pain is worse.

This is why, as far as possible, it's essential to focus on your sleep cycles as a disabled person. If you're worried about your sleep, you can speak to your GP. They may be able to offer treatments for issues affecting your sleep, such as mental health. They might recommend talking therapies, medication, or even a referral to a sleep clinic. But – if you don't feel able to talk to your GP yet – there are several things which you could try yourself to see if they improve your sleep quality.

It's helped me to establish a sleep routine and good sleep habits, alternatively known as 'sleep hygiene'. I always have a warm bath or shower whilst watching something good, then have a warm cup of sleep tea, turn off my phone, and read in bed for an hour or so before going to sleep. You might need to try different things to find out what works for you. It can help to do something relaxing before bed, such as reading a book or listening to relaxing podcasts or music. Especially if you have a lot of stress or anxiety, finding a way to relax before bed is crucial; you could even try some breathing exercises, meditations, or mindfulness exercises to see if they help – more on this shortly. Whilst you're exploring your nighttime routine, it might be a good idea to keep a sleep journal. You could keep information on your bedtime routine, the time you went to bed, how long you slept for, how well you slept, how many times you awoke in the night, your overall mood, and whether you slept during the day. If you're really struggling with your sleep, you could show your journal to your GP or a healthcare professional to work out what's going on for you.

As well as establishing a good sleep routine, there are a few other things you could try. You could make your sleeping area more comfortable. If you're able, it's worth investing in a supportive mattress that suits your needs and the way you sleep. Making a comfortable sleeping area doesn't need to break the bank, though. You might try to make it cooler or warmer by adding a fan or some cosy blankets, respectively. You could try different lighting levels by introducing dimmer lamps that aren't as bright as overhead lights. If noise is a problem, you could try some earplugs. Loop have some great ear plugs designed specifically for sleep, and

Snoozeband have created sleep headphones for if you want to listen to nature sounds or a podcast to block out noise whilst you sleep. You could even try different bedding for comfort or add a weighted blanket – these can be especially useful for those with anxiety and neurodivergent people.

Another thing to think about is your use of electronic devices and their settings, as research has shown that using screens late into the evening can affect your sleep quality.[31][32] Instead, you could try avoiding screens up to two hours before bed or reduce the brightness of your screens by activating the night light setting on your devices. Avoiding stimulating activities such as playing video games before bed can improve your sleep quality too, as can reducing distractions by switching your phone to silent, airplane, or do not disturb mode.

In addition to your use of screens, another thing to consider is your diet and your overall mental and physical health. Avoiding large meals just before bed can help you sleep better. Incorporating some gentle physical exercise – but in a paced way – into your day might help you to sleep better but try not to do this too close to your bedtime. Finding support for any mental health issues, whether its

---

[31] Daneyal Arshad, Usaid Munir Joyia et al. (2021) The adverse impact of excessive smartphone screen-time on sleep quality among young adults: A prospective cohort [Online]. Available at https://pmc.ncbi.nlm.nih.gov/articles/PMC8776263/ (Accessed 8 August 2025).

[32] Liv McMahon. (1 April 2025) Screen time in bed linked to worse sleep, study finds [Online]. Available at https://www.bbc.co.uk/news/articles/cz79jpxzev5o (Accessed 8 August 2025).

medication or therapy, can help with your sleep quality too. Perhaps most importantly, don't force yourself to sleep, as this can only cause more stress and anxiety. Instead, try to do something relaxing before bed or, if you're really struggling to get to sleep, get up and do something calming in a low light until you feel tired and ready for sleep.

Sleep is key for both our mental and physical health, although this can be problematic when you're disabled. But establishing a good routine, practicing sleep hygiene, creating a comfortable sleeping space, and minimising your use of electronic devices before bed can all help to improve your sleep quality. As ever, though, the best thing to do if you have concerns or if you have persistent issues with sleep is to consult a healthcare professional such as your GP, who may be able to refer you to a specialist for further investigations or sleep studies.

Gentle movement and exercise

Another thing which can have a positive impact on both mental and physical health is gentle physical activity and movement. Once again, though, we ought to acknowledge that for those with mental and physical conditions, getting active can be difficult. It might be hard to find the motivation to exercise, or you might have limited mobility due to a physical disability. However, physical activity does not necessarily need to be intensive HIIT workouts but can

231

include any movement your body does that uses energy. This might be as part of your everyday activities, such as cooking, cleaning, getting the shopping, or doing the gardening. You can, then, incorporate movement into your routine just by going about your day as normal. You could still choose to be active by exercising, which is physical activity that we do intentionally. You might exercise to improve a skill, build strength, or as part of social groups like sports clubs.

However you incorporate being active into your day, movement has lots of benefits for our physical and mental wellbeing. It can help with managing stress and anxiety, raising your mood, improving your sleep, or building confidence. Movement can allow us to connect with nature, socialise with others, improve memory and brain functioning, and reduces the risk of developing some long-term conditions such as heart disease. But there may be times when physical activity isn't helpful for our mental health and can even make us feel worse. This might be the case if you don't enjoy the activity that you're doing, if you over-exercise, or if you use exercise as part of an eating disorder or body dysmorphic disorder (BDD). There may alternatively be things which prevent us from being as active as we'd like, including mobility or physical health issues, living in an area with limited safe places to exercise, or not having enough money to engage in the activities we want to pursue.

You might feel frustrated if things don't feel right the first few times you exercise or try a new activity. In such instances, it might help to work with your highs and lows. There are many reasons why you might find it hard to be active at certain times. For me, exercising late tends to affect my sleep, and I struggle to exercise in the morning as I wake up feeling stiff and sore with chronic pain due to my EDS joints. Instead, it's better for me to exercise in the middle of the day. Try to learn when the best time is for *your* body to engage in physical activity and work with it. Be kind to yourself if you can't be as active as you'd like at a particular time. It's always alright to slow down or even take a break. Remind yourself too that it can take time to find an activity that you like, and it might help to keep trying different ones or changing your routine until something sticks. At the same time, it's ok to stop doing an activity that isn't working for you or which you find worsens your mental or physical health. Some people can find it difficult not to compare themselves with others who are more physically active, or who look a certain way. Try instead to set your own goals based on *your* abilities and what you'd like to achieve. Pay attention to what you're doing and how you're feeling, rather than constantly comparing to others.

For certain activities, finances can be a barrier to getting active, especially as adaptive equipment such as sports wheelchairs often cost into the thousands. But there are plenty of ways to reduce such costs. Your local council or leisure centre may have information about discounts available for certain classes and gyms which are accessible. Some GPs may offer social prescriptions for people with mental or physical health conditions, which can include discounted or free exercise programmes at the local gym. The NHS Better Health programme has information on discounts and introductory offers for getting active and the NHS Fitness Studio has workout videos that you can do from home. The NHS 'Couch to 5k' is another free scheme with an app that can introduce you to walking and running, and which can be adapted for those who need mobility aids. Finally, the NHS Active 10 app helps you to track and build up daily walks to get you moving.

In addition to these free resources and classes, there are so many other things you can do to keep as active as you can, even with a disability. A lot of this advice concerns planning how and when you want to be active, as a good plan can help to take the stress and anxiety out of exercising. You might want to think about what you like to do and what your body is able to do, as this will help you to find an enjoyable and safe activity. Consider as well where you want to be active, and whether you want to exercise together with another person or in a group. Choose the environment that you feel most comfortable with, whether that's the gym, the pool, outside in nature, or somewhere else entirely. There are even plenty of physical activities that you can do online at home. You might be content to exercise by yourself, but if you're getting back into exercise or are anxious, it can help to have someone else with you for moral support and to keep you accountable. You could exercise together or virtually via video call.

Getting into an exercise routine can also help with any anxiety around physical activity. By building habits and setting daily targets that you can tick off, you will feel a sense of accomplishment! You could even set a daily reminder on your phone to keep you consistent. If you reward yourself for moving each day, this will help with your motivation and building your confidence. But it's important to set realistic goals and expectations. When you're disabled, it might take longer to build up your fitness than a non-disabled person. Doing too much at first might make you over-tired or throw you into a boom-and-bust cycle, which could put you off exercising once and for all. Instead, it's a good idea to start off slowly and build up to more if you feel comfortable. Remember too that it's ok to adapt activities to your needs and abilities.

When it comes to exercising as a disabled person, you ought to only do what you can and don't push yourself if exercising feels like it's too much at any particular time. Try instead to adapt to how you're feeling; it's perfectly ok to skip a planned activity if your body or mind are not feeling up to it. Remind yourself that any kind of movement is good, and that it doesn't need to be planned sport or exercise to count as being active. You could incorporate other small ways to increase your physical activity into your daily routine, such as getting off the bus a stop or two early and walking the rest of the way if you can. Be gentle with yourself. If you don't manage to do what you were originally planning, that's ok – the key thing is that you've done your best. Perhaps most importantly, if you have any concerns regarding whether an activity will be suitable with your disability, it can help to consult a medical professional such as a GP or physiotherapist, who can then advise on how to exercise safely and how to make sure the activity meets your needs.

Healthy Eating

Some studies have suggested that what we eat, and drink, can affect how we feel.[33] However, it can be difficult to think about our diet and healthy eating when you're struggling with your mental or physical health. Even if you're having a hard time with your health, though, there are a few key things we can do to improve our diet, if you're able to do so. However, these things are not the case for those with feeding tubes or who are on special or restricted diets due to gastric conditions.

Blood sugar levels can have a direct impact on the way you're feeling. If your level is lower than usual, you might feel tired, irritable, or depressed. Regularly eating foods which release energy slowly can keep your blood sugar levels balanced. These foods include things like wholegrain bread, nuts and seeds, brown pasta, and brown rice. If you have diabetes, though, you should speak to

---

[33] British Nutrition Foundation. (2025) Food and your brain: Eating for a better mood [Online]. Available at https://www.nutrition.org.uk/nutrition-for/food-and-the-brain/ (Accessed 8 August 2025).

your GP or diabetes nurse before making any changes to your diet which could affect your blood sugar levels.

Eating different fruits and vegetables can add a good range of nutrients to your diet. These nutrients help to keep us mentally and physically healthy. Frozen, tinned, dried, and juiced fruits and vegetables all count towards your 5 a day too, if these options are more accessible to you. Diets that are higher in protein can also support your mental health. Protein contains amino acids, which your brain needs to produce chemicals called neurotransmitters, to regulate your thoughts and feelings. Protein is in foods like legumes, nuts and seeds, milk, fish, eggs, cheese, and soya products. Your brain needs certain healthy fatty acids too, such as omega-3 and omega-6, to keep it working well. These healthy fats can be found in nuts and seeds, avocado, and oily fish.

Sometimes, your gut can really reflect your mood. If you're stressed or anxious, this could make your digestion speed up or slow down, leading to problems with digestion and appetite. It can be difficult to eat well when you have poor mental or physical health anyway, as food and eating can be triggering for many. There are a few things you could try, though. If you're able, try to write down how food is making you feel throughout each day. This can help you to work out which foods make you feel emotionally or physically better or worse, which keep you awake or give you energy, and which foods affect your sleep, as these are all key areas for your mental health.

If you're finding cooking and eating physically difficult with a disability, there are a few things you can try. Planning ahead when you're feeling well can help to take the stress out of those times when you're feeling worse. You could make some extra meals to store in the fridge or freezer for when you have flare-ups, or stock up on some staple ingredients so you can always make a tasty meal quickly. Writing a list of easy-to-make and affordable meals can help too to reduce decision-fatigue. If going to the supermarket and collecting your shopping is physically difficult for you, look for services where your shopping gets delivered to your door, saving time and energy. You could instead try to accept help from others. This can be difficult for many disabled people, especially if they're adamant about maintaining their independence. But accepting help with practical things such as fetching the shopping or cooking and eating a meal together can make the whole process feel less daunting for you and can help with any anxiety or physical fatigue you're experiencing.

Food preparation is another key area which people with disabilities or mental health conditions might find difficult. To make preparation easier, it can help to wash up or put dishes into the dishwasher as you go. Washing up bit by bit can help you to pace your energy and can make you feel less overwhelmed by the task at hand. If you're really struggling with the washing up due to a flare-up, it might be worth looking at disposable plates, cutlery, and paper towels for a short while. Another top tip is to make food all in one pot or dish. This reduces the amount of equipment you need to use and clean; slow-cookers can be especially helpful for one-pot dishes, especially as all you need to do is put your ingredients into the pot in the morning and it will slowly cook you a delicious meal as the day passes! You could equally invest in kitchen aids that will make food preparation less taxing for you. Things like L-shaped knives, lightweight measuring jugs, liquid level indicators, and even air-fryers are all great pieces of adaptive equipment you could try. Finally, try pre-chopped or frozen fruits and vegetables in your dishes. This can reduce the amount of food preparation you have to do and frozen versions of fruit and vegetables are often cheaper and more accessible than the fresh varieties.

Drinking Enough Water

If you live with a mental health condition, you may not have the energy or the motivation to drink a lot of fluids. But if you become dehydrated, this can make it much harder for you to concentrate and think clearly. Water, tea, juices, and smoothies can all help you to feel hydrated but be careful of those which might contain high levels of sugar or caffeine, which could affect how you feel in a negative way. Some people find it useful to track their daily fluid intake by writing it down, setting a reminder on their phone, or getting a water bottle which has measurements on it to tell you how much you ought to drink and how often.

Reaching out to others

If you're struggling with your mental or physical health, it can help to talk to someone you trust about how you are feeling. They might be able to help you find out more information, discuss your options or come to appointments with you, help practically with everyday tasks, and give support and encouragement.

A member of your family or someone from your friendship circle is often the one trusted person you want to discuss things with. Sometimes, though, it can be difficult to talk to your family or friends about how you're feeling; you might be anxious about upsetting someone you are close with, or you might feel nervous about what people will think and how it will affect your relationship. At times, I've struggled to talk to my family and friends as I've desperately wanted to resolve things on my own, and I didn't want to be a burden on my loved ones, especially with my disability. I was worried what they might think of me and how I was going to express what was going through my head.

There are some tips that can help here. Find a method of communication that feels right for you as this will help to reduce your anxiety around the conversation; this could be via phone or video chat, meeting someone face-to-face, or you could even write down how you feel in a text message or letter. If you are meeting in person, or having a phone or video call, find a suitable time and place to call or meet, where it is quiet, and where you feel comfortable. You could practice what you want to say beforehand or make some notes on the key things that you want to express to your loved one. It can help to be open and honest, and just explain how you're feeling and how it's affecting your life so that others can better understand what you're going through. Depending on your relationship, you could suggest things that your loved one could do to help you through this tough time. You might just want your friend or family member to listen and offer emotional support, or to practically help you; letting them know what kind of support you need is key to them being able to help you in the ways that you need.

It's important to stress that you ought not to expect too much from one conversation with your loved one. They may understand you instantly and be there to offer you the support that you need. However, mental health conditions can take some time for others to fully understand, and some people may be shocked at first to hear the struggles you're experiencing. Remember that this is new information you're presenting to your loved one, so they need space to respond emotionally too. Give them some time to process what you have told them, and plan to come back to the conversation later to review things. If you do not feel comfortable talking to a friend or family member, it's important to still reach out to someone who can help, whether that is a GP or another healthcare professional. You could instead reach out to a mental health service in your local area or a national charity such as Mind, Samaritans, or the National

Suicide Prevention Helpline UK. You can find details of some organisations that might be helpful below.[34]

Mind support line: 0300 102 1234.

Open 9:00am – 6:00pm, Monday to Friday except bank holidays.

Samaritans: 116 126 or emails jo@samaritans.org.

Open 24 hours a day, 365 days a year.

SANEline: 0300 304 7000.

Open 4:30pm to 10:00pm every day.

Campaign Against Living Miserably (CALM): 0800 58 58 58 or use the CALM webchat service.

Open 5:00pm to 12:00am every day.

Switchboard: 0300 330 0630 or email chris@switchboard.lgbt.

For people who identify as LGBTQIA+. Open 10:00am to 10:00pm every day.

---

[34] Please note that all information was correct at time of publication [31 October 2025]. Please always check each organisation's website for the most up-to-date information in cases of changes to these details.

Spending time in nature

Spending time in green space or bringing nature into your everyday life can benefit both your mental and your physical wellbeing. Growing your own fruits, vegetables, or flowers, exercising outdoors, or being around animals can have lots of positive effects, such as reducing feelings of anxiety, depression, or stress, and improving your mood. Spending time outdoors can also connect you with your local community, helping you to meet new people and combatting feelings of loneliness. When you feel more connected to nature, studies have shown that this helps with mental health problems such as anxiety and depression.[35] Recent research into ecotherapy has suggested that being outside in nature can help with mild to moderate depression, and that being in natural light can positively improve seasonal affective disorder (SAD).[36]

However, connecting with the natural world can be difficult when you have a mental health condition or disability. Not all outdoor spaces are accessible to people with mobility issues, and if you are anxious or depressed, you may worry or lack the motivation

---

[35] University of York. (16 April 2025) Nature-based activity is effective therapy for anxiety and depression, study shows [Online]. Available at https://www.york.ac.uk/news-and-events/news/2025/research/nature-based-activity-therapy-anxiety-depression/ (Accessed 8 August 2025).

[36] Mind: Norfolk and Waveney. (2025) Nature and Mental Health [Online]. Available at https://www.norfolkandwaveneymind.org.uk/nature-mental-health#:~:text=For%20example%2C%20research%20into%20ecotherapy,Related%20Links%20&%20Resources (Accessed 8 August 2025).

243

to access natural spaces. There are nevertheless many small ways in which we can bring a bit more of nature into our everyday lives, even with a disability. Start small, as even spending small amounts of time in nature can boost your mood. You could try starting with either five minutes being outside or in your home looking out at nature and then build up gradually to help you pace your energy and activity. Doing things which work for you and which you find relaxing can encourage you to spend more time in nature too. You might enjoy watching birds or maybe being near water or in a forest; you might prefer walking in nature, or you might prefer sitting and observing the nature around you. By doing activities which you enjoy, you'll be more motivated to stick to your routine and introduce time in nature into your day in small, relaxing stints.

'Nature' does not have to mean going far afield to connect with the natural world around you. Nature is everywhere, even in busy towns and cities – you only need to look. You might want to take a stroll around your local area and just notice the trees, birds, insects, the weather, and the sky. You could look for local green spaces too. Your council may have information about which nature reserves are near to you, and which are accessible or free to visit. You might want to use walking apps like Go Jaunty to find local nature walks to you. The Wildlife Trust, the National Trust, and the Outdoor Guide are all great places to start to find information on accessible and nearby green spaces you might want to visit.

Another option to incorporate nature into your daily life is to bring it indoors. You could buy flowers or potted plants to display around your house or flat, or you might collect natural materials such as stones, crystals, or dried flowers to display. You might even take photos of your favourite places in nature and hang them on your wall to contemplate each time you go past. Alternatively, you could listen to natural sound podcasts on Spotify or other streaming services or watch videos of nature. This can help to make the natural world more accessible to those with disabilities, especially those who cannot leave their homes. If you have a balcony, allotment space, or back garden, another possibility is to take up gardening. There are many things like miniature greenhouses and raised trugs which can take advantage of limited space, and which can make gardening more accessible when you have a disability. There are, then, lots of ways to connect with nature, whether that's by spending time outside in the natural world or whether you try to bring a bit of it into your indoor space. Both ways are beneficial for our mental and physical health, so there's no right or wrong here. The most important thing is to choose the way that is accessible and sustainable for your needs.

Practicing gratitude

Practicing gratitude is a great way to improve your wellbeing, as it helps to train your brain to notice and appreciate the little things. Spending time on gratitude each day can increase your happiness,

245

life satisfaction, and even your overall health whilst decreasing anxiety and depression. It is therefore a powerful practice to cultivate.

Mental health conditions all concern the content of *what* we think and the process of *how* we think, both of which impact our anxiety and depression. Ruminating too much on our thoughts can pull you out of the present moment and can add to these anxious and depressed feelings. Gratitude counters these thinking habits. But when you're stuck in a spiral of anxiety and depression, it can be difficult to tap into gratitude and you can easily get stuck in negative thinking patterns instead. When this happens, challenge your mind to find something in that one moment for which you are grateful, which will bring your mind back to the present. Indeed, studies show that a single act of thoughtful gratitude produces an immediate 10% increase in happiness and a 35% reduction in depressive symptoms.[37] But for gratitude to be effective, we need to practice it repeatedly.

To cultivate practicing gratitude, at the end of each day, I tend to write down in my diary three things that have happened throughout the day that I'm grateful for; these don't need to be grand gestures but can be simple things like a colleague making me a cup of tea

---

[37] Mental Health First Aid. (26 November 2024) Cultivating Gratitude in the Workplace – Turning Challenges into Triumphs [Online]. Available at https://www.mentalhealthfirstaid.org/2024/11/cultivating-gratitude-workplace-challenges-triumphs/ (Accessed 8 August 2025).

246

when I was feeling down. Writing down these thoughts or saying them aloud reinforces them and helps you to stay positive during difficult times. You could keep a gratitude journal either as a written diary or as a note on your phone and write down a certain number of things that you're thankful for each day. You could even write these out on slips of paper and put them into a gratitude jar; you can then draw thoughts from the jar to remind you of all the good things when you are struggling.

Another key aspect of practising gratitude is to celebrate small victories, even if it's something like getting out of bed on a bad day. To help build the habit of practising gratitude, you could pick a time each week where you'll reflect on things that went right in the week and celebrate any small wins that you've had. Practising mindfulness can also help when it comes to gratitude, as it allows you to pay attention to the present moment and notice life's small pleasures. Finally, you could try expressing your thanks to someone for something they have done for you. Even if it's something small, or something that usually goes unnoticed, such as saying thank you to the cleaners at work for keeping your work environment clean, tidy, and pleasant for you to work in. Saying thank you to someone else and seeing their reaction is infectious, and can often make us feel brighter, even if it has been a hard day. Practising gratitude has many benefits for our mental health and wellbeing. It reduces stress and anxiety, increases happiness, improves relationships, boosts self-esteem, and counteracts depression. Incorporating gratitude into your life doesn't need to be difficult – just start by noticing one thing you're thankful for right now.

Mindfulness and breathing

If you are disabled or have a chronic illness – especially one which causes chronic pain – you've likely heard about mindfulness from condition or pain management courses. But it's not always clear what exactly it is. Mindfulness has its roots in Buddhism and meditation. It is a way of drawing our attention to the present moment without judgement; you just take notice and be aware of your mind, body, and surroundings in that moment. Amongst its other benefits, mindfulness can help you to become more self-aware; feel calmer and less stressed; choose how to respond to difficult, anxious, or worrying thoughts and feelings; be kinder to yourself; and manage chronic pain.

Mindfulness works by drawing your focus to the present moment and away from other thoughts and feelings. It allows you to notice how your thoughts come and go and what your body is trying to tell you. Mindfulness can help those with chronic pain to manage this by highlighting that pain is just one part of their experience. Research has shown that practicing mindfulness improves depression, anxiety, coping ability, and acceptance.[38] It

---

[38] NHS. (2025) Mindfulness [Online]. Available at https://www.nhs.uk/mental-health/self-help/tips-and-

can also have a moderate and lasting effect in reducing pain intensity in those with chronic pain. Extensive research has been conducted on the effectiveness of mindfulness for chronic pain management. It is increasingly showing that practising mindfulness daily can reduce a person's experience of chronic pain and help them to manage negative or worrisome thoughts about their pain.[39]

Just like any skill, mindfulness requires practice and patience. Thankfully, there are a lot of relaxation techniques and exercises out there, many of which you can do by yourself and without any equipment. There are plenty of guided mindfulness exercises that are available for free online. Not every exercise will work for everyone and, if that is the case for you, don't worry – simply try another exercise until one sticks. Below are some exercises which have helped me before and which you could try. More information and guided meditations can be found online, and the NHS's *Every Mind Matters* site has an audio guide for relaxing your body:

- **Mindful eating.** Paying attention to taste, texture, and the appearance of what you eat.

---

support/mindfulness/#:~:text=Studies%20show%20that%20mindfulness%20can,can%20make%20them%20feel%20worse. (Accessed 8 August 2025).

[39] J Kabat-Zinn, L Lipworth & R Burney. (1985) The clinical use of mindfulness meditation for the self-regulation of chronic pain [Online]. Available at https://pubmed.ncbi.nlm.nih.gov/3897551/#:~:text=Abstract,chronic%20pain%20control%20is%20discussed. (Accessed 8 August 2025).

- **Mindful walking.** Focusing on the movement and sensations in your body as you go on a walk, maybe in nature or a relaxing setting.

- **Mindful body scan.** Find somewhere quiet and comfortable where you won't be interrupted and lie or sit down. Close your eyes. Slowly move your focus through different parts of your body, starting at your head and moving to your toes. Note how each body part feels and any sensations you experience. You could try tensing and then relaxing each part of your body as you go for deeper relaxation. It can help to match this to your breathing; tense your muscles as you take a deep breath in, then relax as you breathe out.

- **Mindful colouring.** There are plenty of mindful adult colouring books available online or in shops, as well as free printable images for colouring online. Focus on the colours and on the sensation of your pencil or pen against the paper.

- **Active relaxation.** Relaxation doesn't just mean sitting or lying on your sofa. Gentle movement and exercise can be relaxing if you choose carefully. You could take a relaxing walk, attend a yoga or Pilates class, or try some seated exercises. The last suggestion might help to integrate movement into your day if you're busy at work or if you're a mobility aid user. The NHS has guidance on seated exercises you can try.

- **Drawing calming circles.** This exercise helps distract from any anxiety and gives you an outlet for your emotions. You will need a table or desk, blank paper, and something to draw or colour with, such as pens, pencils, or crayons. Sit comfortably and take up your paper and pen. Draw a circle on the paper that fills most of the page, it doesn't have to be neat. Then keep drawing. You could keep going over your original circle, or fill it with a pattern, but try not to let your pencil leave the page. You don't need to create a finished picture, just keep going. Take time as you go to focus on what you're drawing and the sensations in your mind and body. Once you have been drawing for a few minutes, try using a different colour or pattern, and keep drawing until you feel calm and relaxed.

- **Take a mindful moment in nature.** As we've already seen, spending time in nature has been found to reduce stress, anxiety, and depression. Find yourself a green space to sit in, whether indoors or outdoors. Take a deep breath and start exploring slowly. Try not to focus on getting somewhere in particular. Focus on any movement your make and notice the ground underneath you and the surrounding nature. Listen to the sounds around you; is there birdsong or can you hear the wind rustling the leaves of trees? Take note of any smells, such as flowers or freshly cut grass. Keep exploring and noting what your senses take in until you feel calmer.

- **Connect with your senses.** If you are feeling stressed, overwhelmed, or panicked, connecting with your five senses can help to ground you in the present moment. You can do this exercise anywhere and anytime, as you just need yourself. Take a deep breath and settle into your surroundings. Once you feel ready, look around you and notice five things that you can see. You can name these in

251

your head, write them on paper or say them aloud. Next name four things you can touch or feel around you. Then name three things you can hear around you. You can then name two things that you can smell around you, and finally, name one thing that you can taste.

Relaxation and mindfulness can help to give you some mental respite from intrusive worrying thoughts, feelings, and anxiety. There are a lot of techniques and exercises out there, many of which you can simply do by yourself in a comfortable space. I have practiced mindfulness for several years now, both for anxiety and for my chronic pain. It has helped me to shift my perspective and see my pain as passing in a transient moment. But just like any skill, mindfulness didn't come easy to me at first and I had to put in a lot of practice to get better at it, even if it became frustrating at times! So here are a few tips that I learned along the way that I hope will help you too:

- **Pay attention.** Focus on sensations, the things that you can see, hear, smell, touch, and taste.

- **Take notice.** When your mind wanders – which it is natural for it to do – simply notice where your thoughts have drifted without any judgement. Some people find it helpful to name and acknowledge the thoughts or feelings that they have. Then just gently guide your thoughts back to the present moment.

- **Be aware and accepting.** Notice the emotions you feel and the sensations you are feeling in your body as you practice mindfulness. You do not need to try and get rid of these feelings and sensations. Instead, acknowledge them and accept them with friendly curiosity, and without judgement.

- **Be kind to yourself.** Mindfulness can be difficult, and it is natural for our minds to wander. For some, practising mindfulness may feel decidedly *un*natural. Try not to be critical or judgemental of yourself or your thoughts and feelings. When you notice that your mind is wandering, just gently bring your focus back to the present moment and to the exercise at hand.

As disabled people, mindfulness can be a powerful tool in your kit for dealing with depression, anxiety, stress, and chronic pain. It can improve our ability to cope with stressful thoughts and situations, as well as your quality of life and sleep quality. Mindfulness is therefore a handy skill to acquire to look after our mental health and wellbeing.

Journalling

Journalling is the act of keeping a record of your personal thoughts, feelings, insights, reflections, and more and so it can be a useful tool for self-care and wellbeing. Journalling provides a safe space to express your thoughts and emotions without judgement, and can help you to process them, gain clarity, and identify patterns. Writing about events that you have found stressful or depressing can offload the weight of them and reduce your stress levels. Journalling can further allow you to analyse situations and problems more

253

objectively, weigh the pros and cons, and try out possible solutions. It caan similarly be a useful tool to note down and track your symptoms day to day to identify triggers and learn better ways of managing them.

The practice of journalling can help your mental health and wellbeing in many ways. Writing about your feelings is linked to reduced mental distress. Researchers found that those with various medical conditions and anxiety who wrote for 15 minutes, three days a week, over a 12-week period, had increased feelings of wellbeing and fewer symptoms of anxiety and depression after a month.[40] Journalling about an emotional event can help you to break the cycle of over-thinking and brooding over what happened; you can instead analyse the situation and try out possible solutions. Journalling can also regulate our emotions. Brain scans of people who wrote about their feelings demonstrated that they were able to control their emotions better than those who wrote about a neutral experience.[41] Among its many other benefits, journalling can

---

[40] Cobb Collaborative. (2025) Journaling as a Recovery and Resilience Building Tool [Online]. Available at https://www.cobbcollaborative.org/journaling-as-a-recovery-and-resilience-building-tool#:~:text=In%20a%20study%2C%20researchers%20found,the%2012%20weeks%20of%20journaling. (Accessed 8 August 2025).

[41] Ian Sample. (15 February 2009) Keeping a diary makes you happier [Online]. Available at https://www.theguardian.com/science/2009/feb/15/psychology-usa#:~:text=Those%20who%20wrote%20about%20an%20emotional%20experi

encourage us to open up. Writing privately about an upsetting or stressful event can encourage us to reach out for emotional support from others, thereby supporting our mental health and wellbeing.

When I went through a pain management course for my chronic pain, my healthcare professional gave me a journal and asked me to write in it each day, no matter how small, even if it was just one word to sum up the day. It might be a surprise to hear that journalling did not come naturally to me – yes, even though I wrote a whole PhD and this entire book! At first, I struggled to think what to write and was worried about sounding overly emotional. As time went by, though, I found myself opening up. I began to write more and more, letting my pen and mind wander and diving deeper into my emotions. Journalling essentially helped me to better analyse my problems and to express more clearly and concisely how I was feeling with my therapist. Whilst my early journalling entries focused on my experience and emotions around my chronic pain, I continue to keep a journal to this day and my entries now centre around all sorts of feelings and issues that come up in my daily life. Without my journal, I know that I would not be as far along in my journey with chronic pain as I am now, especially after the onset of

---

ence,neural%20activity%20linked%20to%20strong%20emotional%20feelings. (Accessed 8 August 2025).

Complex Regional Pain Syndrome, which truly turned my world upside down.

When it came to getting started with journalling, I most certainly did not take to it like a duck to water. Below are some tips for starting off and building up your journalling practice, which I hope will come in handy for you, if you decide to give journalling a try:

- **Choose your medium.** You could select the traditional notebook and pen, or you might prefer a digital app or document on your computer. Choose a format that you find inviting and convenient, and one that you're likely to enjoy using regularly, as this will help to maintain your motivation to journal.

- **Create a routine.** Find a time of the day which suits your schedule and dedicate it to writing in your journal. It doesn't need to be long – even five or ten minutes a day will help. A consistent routine can help to incorporate journalling into your life and build it into a habit.

- **Find a comfortable space.** Choose a quiet spot where you can get into the flow and write without interruptions. Find a place where you feel at ease as this will help you to start writing.

- **Write regularly.** Aim to write in your journal daily if you can, even if it is only a word or a few sentences. Regular writing helps to develop the habit of journalling and makes it a core part of your mental health, wellbeing, and self-care routine. Consistency matters!

- **Let go of judgement and be authentic.** Approach your journalling with an open mind. Remember that this is your private space, so let go of any concerns about grammar, spelling, or negative self-talk. Write freely, honestly, and authentically, expressing whatever comes to mind. The more honest you are with yourself, the more beneficial that journalling will be for you; don't hide your true feelings away!

- **Dive deeper into your emotions.** Instead of just noting down events, focus on exploring your thoughts and feelings about them. This kind of deeper exploration can provide insights into your emotional triggers and help you to manage your emotional responses to events more effectively.

- **Be mindful.** By incorporating tenets of mindfulness, you can turn your journalling into a meditative practice that helps you focus your thoughts and feelings on the present moment. Observing your thoughts without judgement can enhance your self-awareness and emotional regulation.

- **Use prompts.** Some days, you may be completely stuck on what to write about. Don't judge yourself, this is perfectly normal. To help you keep writing, you could try journalling prompts, which can spark creativity and provide a structured way to explore different aspects of your experiences and emotions.

- **Reflect on your progress.** You might want to take time to look back on earlier journal entries to get a sense of your personal growth and progress. It's important to remind ourselves of how far we've come and celebrate the small wins!

- **Journal for gratitude.** To really enhance your mental health and wellbeing, dedicate part of your journalling to practicing gratitude, as this can improve your mood and overall sense of wellbeing. Gratitude journalling has been linked to reductions in negative thoughts and a more positive outlook on life.

- **Explore different journalling styles.** As you get more confident in your journalling, you might want to experiment with different journalling styles to find the one you prefer, and which best suits your needs. Whether its bullet journalling, stream of consciousness, or structured reflective writing, different styles can offer new perspectives and benefits.

Journalling can be a useful way to explore your thoughts and feelings, and to improve your overall mental health and wellbeing. There are so many different styles of journalling you can try, so just test them out until you find one which works for you.

Medication and professional help

One of the most important ways that you can support your mental health and wellbeing is to reach out for professional help, whether that's from a therapist or a healthcare professional such as your GP or a specialist. Seeking help is often the first step towards getting and staying well. Many people feel unsure where to start and are apprehensive about reaching out for help. They may wonder

258

instead whether they should just try to handle things on their own, especially if they're worried about being a burden to someone else. But it's always a good idea to ask for help, even if you're not sure whether you are experiencing a specific mental health problem. There are lots of options for support out there, but you might find some are more suitable for you or more easily accessible than others.

For many of us, our GP is one of the first places we go to when we feel unwell. Your doctor is there to help you with your mental as well as your physical health. Your GP might be able to make a diagnosis of a specific mental health problem, or might offer you support or treatments, including medication and talking therapies such as Cognitive Behavioural Therapy (CBT). Your doctor might also refer you to a mental health specialist or recommend local support options. Trained therapists and counsellors can provide a range of different therapies either privately or through the NHS.

There are many ways that you can find a therapist who suits your needs. You might be eligible for some therapy sessions for free on the NHS. These services are usually called talking therapies or psychological wellbeing services. In some areas of the UK, you can actually refer yourself for NHS counselling, or your GP can refer you too. There are some other providers of free therapy in the UK. Your local library, GP surgery, or community centre are all great places to find out about the affordable services where you live. Some mental health charities run free helplines, listening services, and peer support groups for those experiencing mental health difficulties. Some of these charities include Mind UK, Anxiety UK, Mental Health Matters, or Cruse Bereavement Support.

If you are in employment, your workplace might have an Employee Assistance Programme (EAP). These services tend to offer some free counselling sessions, and you can usually access these without needing to go through your line manager or HR. If you are a student at college or university, your institution should have a free student counselling service, and you should be able to access it without going through your personal tutor if you would prefer them not to be involved. Finally, there is private therapy available in the UK, and you might want to go private if you can't get the therapy that you need from the NHS. If you are exploring going privately, you can try looking on the following directories for a therapist:

- The Counselling Directory.

- The British Association for Counselling and Psychotherapy (BACP).

- The UK Council for Psychotherapy (UKCP).

- The Human Givens Institute Directory.

- The National Counselling and Psychotherapy Society (NCPS).

- The Black, African and Asian Therapy Network (BAATN).

- The Muslim Counsellor and Psychotherapist Network (MCAPN).

- Pink Therapy for therapists from the LGBTQIA+ community.

If you are struggling with your mental health and wellbeing, it's always a good idea to reach out for help. But when you are struggling, it can feel incredibly daunting, overwhelming, and anxiety-inducing to even think about reaching out to a professional. If you are worried about approaching a healthcare or other professional, it might help to reach out to a friend or family member first; they could then accompany and support you in seeking professional help. When I was struggling the most with my chronic pain, to the point that it was severely affecting my mental health and wellbeing, I was worried about talking to my GP about it. I thought that they might be dismissive or not believe that my pain was that bad and having such an impact on my life. Talking to my mum first helped me to better articulate how I was feeling. When it came to speaking with my GP, my mum came with me for moral support and helped to emphasise just how much my chronic pain was affecting my mental health and overall wellbeing. Having a supportive person in the room can be immensely helpful, as they might think of questions to ask your healthcare professional that you had not even considered, or they could help by taking notes. If you can reach out to someone supportive in your life first, it can help you so much in reaching out for professional support.

Dealing with chronic pain

Now that we've looked at several ways you can help to manage your mental health and wellbeing, it's worth talking about chronic pain. For me, chronic pain is a huge part of my life, especially due to my Complex Regional Pain Syndrome (CRPS). Usually, when you injure yourself – such as spraining your ankle – it hurts. So, you go to the doctor, and they strap it up. You know it will hurt for a short while, but that it will get better, and the pain will stop. When you have chronic pain, you know that there is no endpoint for your pain, that doctors will rarely be able to help, and sometimes there is no injury or cause to attribute the pain to – it just happens. Living in constant pain takes so much mental strength to face, knowing that every day afterwards will be the same with your pain. Living with chronic pain can be an incredibly frustrating and isolating experience, then, particularly if those around you do not understand what it's like to be constantly in pain.

It is worth noting as well that women suffer from chronic pain disproportionately in comparison to men.[42] Women are more likely to develop chronic pain from rheumatic and musculoskeletal conditions, as well as experiencing the chronic pain arising from gynaecological conditions such as endometriosis or vaginismus.

---

[42] Nuffield: Women's & Reproductive Health. (2025) Pain in Women [Online]. Available at https://www.wrh.ox.ac.uk/research/pain-in-women#:~:text=Women%20suffer%20with%20almost%20all,with%20diseases%20such%20as%20endometriosis. (Accessed 8 August 2025).

Despite the higher prevalence of chronic pain in women, many remain untreated; this is perhaps due to the long history of medical gaslighting of women's pain, whereby their pain was either dismissed or attributed solely to a psychological cause. It also does not help that, for many decades, research into chronic pain has focused predominantly on male subjects, meaning that treatment recommendations were based on the male experience of chronic pain, further excluding women.[43] When we talk about chronic pain, then, we ought to be aware of these disparities in the treatment of women's pain, which sadly persist in our society today.

Whatever the source of your chronic pain, it can feel all-consuming as it affects every part of your life: your relationships, your hobbies, your work or education, your sleep, and your mental and physical wellbeing, to name but a few. For some, chronic pain can be so intense that it prevents them from doing the things they would really love to do, such as working a job, socialising with friends, or pursuing hobbies. There have certainly been times in my life when chronic pain has left me isolated and frustrated. When I was eighteen, my pain was so intense that it left me confined to bed for months. I had to interrupt my studies at university, nor was I able to take up work or really socialise with my friends. My boyfriend

---

[43] The Lancet: Rheumatology. (2024) Time to listen to women about their pain [Online]. Available at https://www.thelancet.com/journals/lanrhe/article/PIIS2665-9913(24)00126-7/fulltext#:~:text=Every%20day%2C%20millions%20of%20women,chronic%20pain%20is%20still%20scarce. (Accessed 8 August 2025).

would often just come to my house and sit with me as I lay silently in bed and tried to sleep through the worst of the pain. I was so lucky at this time to have a supportive family and partner, but I still felt isolated and lost many friends during that period of intense pain. My friends were all at university, leading exciting lives and they could not relate to what I was experiencing or to living life from my bed. Chronic pain left me feeling incredibly lonely and frustrated that my life seemed to be lagging behind whilst all my friends were moving forwards.

If you are experiencing similar situations with chronic pain, please know that you are not alone. Many of us in the disability community know what it's like to live in pain without respite. If your chronic pain is affecting your physical or mental wellbeing, it's worth reaching out to a healthcare professional to see what support might be available in your local area. There are techniques you can learn that can help with chronic pain too. Once again, I am not a medical expert on managing chronic pain. But as someone who lives with various types of chronic pain, there are some tips and tricks that I've picked up along the way which have made a considerable difference to my pain levels, especially when I've been struggling with my mental health and wellbeing too. Here are a few for you to think about, which I hope will be helpful:

- **Practice breathing exercises.** Focusing on your breathing can distract you from your pain levels by drawing your attention elsewhere. Learning different breathing techniques can help you to distract from pain and feel calmer anywhere and anytime. There are plenty of breathing exercises that you can learn for free from videos online.

- **Regular gentle movement.** Gentle movement can help to ease chronic pain by getting your muscles stretching and your joints moving. Try to work with your body to gradually increase the amount of movement in your daily life, whilst making sure that you are still pacing within your energy budget. You could consider something gentle like yoga, Pilates, or Tai Chi. Once you've built up your exercise tolerance, you could try some of the adaptive sports we looked at in chapter three. As always, if you are concerned about incorporating movement into your daily life with chronic pain, talk to your GP or a healthcare professional about how you can do this safely and in a paced way.

- **Participate in activities that are meaningful to you.** The body's natural feel-good chemicals, endorphins, help to relieve chronic pain. They are activated by exercise, relaxation techniques, and enjoyable experiences. By setting aside time each day for a simple activity which you either find calming or enjoyable, you'll be stimulating your mind and body to release endorphins. Chapter three contains a list of pain-friendly and energy-conscious activities which you could explore if you're at a loss for what to do.

- **Engage in mindfulness techniques.** As we've seen above, practising mindfulness can be beneficial for our overall mental health and wellbeing. It can help those with chronic pain to learn

265

how to better manage their pain levels. Practising mindfulness on a daily basis has been shown to reduce and have a lasting effect on chronic pain intensity, to the point that some people are able to either reduce or eliminate their use of pain medications.[44] If you're looking for mindful activities to try, look earlier in this chapter or search amongst the many free mindfulness meditations and practices available online.

- **Pace your activities.** As we've seen earlier in this chapter, pacing largely helps to manage fatigue levels, but it can help with chronic pain management too. If you experience chronic pain, using pacing techniques can allow you to gradually build up your activity whilst managing your pain levels and ensuring you take plenty of rest breaks to ease your pain. If you're interested in finding out more about pacing techniques, read the section on pacing earlier in this chapter or conduct your own research online.

- **Practice good sleep habits.** Getting enough good-quality sleep is key to managing your pain. When you cannot sleep due to pain, your pain gets worse during the day, which ends up in a vicious cycle of pain leading to no sleep, and no sleep leading to increased

---

[44] Lori Sodeman. (2024) Use mindfulness to cope with pain [Online]. Available at https://www.mayoclinichealthsystem.org/hometown-health/speaking-of-health/use-mindfulness-to-cope-with-chronic-pain#:~:text=Managing%20chronic%20pain%20with%20mindfulness,reduce%20depression%20and%20anxiety%20symptoms. (Accessed 8 August 2025).

pain. The tips that we've looked at earlier in this chapter can help you to get enough good-quality sleep and control your pain levels.

- **Stay connected to your support system.** While it's important to take time for yourself and to focus on your own self-care, having family and friends who care about you is important for managing chronic pain. Although you may want to be left alone during flare-ups, learning to lean in to support from others can help chronic pain feel even a little bit more manageable. There may be practical tasks your loved ones can help with, or it might be enough for them to just be there to listen and provide emotional support for what you're going through. If you want tips on how to build your support network after acquiring a disability, then head to chapter four.

- **Join a support group.** Joining a support group can help you to meet others who experience chronic pain and who will understand what you're going through. You might learn management tips or ways of accessing support from other members too. There is a lot of self-help advice available from various organisations that support people with chronic pain and which run support groups. Action on Pain, the British Pain Society, Pain Concern, and Pain Support are but a few you could explore.

- **Call a helpline.** Even if you do not want to join a support group, it can sometimes help to talk to others who live in chronic pain and who intrinsically understand what you're going through. Pain Concern, Action on Pain, Versus Arthritis, and Burning Nights all have telephone helplines staffed by people with chronic pain. They are sometimes able to put you in touch with local patient support groups, if this is something you want to explore.

- **OTC and prescription medications.** Over the counter (OTC) and prescription medications can help in the management of chronic pain. Research suggests that, on average, medications can achieve a 30% reduction in pain. There are many kinds of pain medications that are available, such as NSAIDs or anti-inflammatories, non-opioid analgesics, opioids, gabapentinoids, and anti-depressants. You can explore with your GP or healthcare professional which medication(s) might be the most effective for you. Unfortunately, there can be a stigma around chronic pain patients taking pain medications – particularly opioids – and this can potentially impact on your mental health and wellbeing. However, if medications help to relieve and manage your pain, try to ignore what other people think and instead focus on what's best for *you* and your pain management. I must now take several medications for my health conditions and have been on the receiving end of stigma because of this. But these medications help me to function and live a fulfilling life – it doesn't matter what other people think, what matters is what works for *you* and *your* pain.

- **Find ways to distract yourself from the pain.** When you focus on your pain, especially if it worries you or you find it distressing, it can make the pain worse. Distraction can be a great technique for managing chronic pain. Find an activity which keeps you busy and which consumes your thoughts, so that you are thinking about things besides your pain. You might not be able to avoid pain entirely, but by using distraction, you can keep it from taking control of your life. If you need any suggestions on adapted or energy-conscious activities which might help, check out chapter three.

- **Talking therapies.** Living in constant pain can make you feel tired, anxious, depressed, frustrated, and isolated and this can make the pain even worse. Living with chronic pain is not easy and some people find it useful to get help from a psychologist through talking therapies to learn how to better deal with the emotions that are linked to their pain. If you want to explore this option, you can either look for a therapist privately or ask your GP or healthcare provider to refer you for NHS support.

- **Pain clinics and management programmes.** If you're having difficulty managing your pain, you can ask your doctor or healthcare professional for a referral to a specialist pain clinic or programme. Pain clinics offer a wide range of treatment options and support, often adopting a biopsychosocial approach to pain management. This describes a model of healthcare support that considers the biological, psychological, and social factors that contribute to a person's health. Pain clinics therefore aim to support you to develop self-help skills to control and relieve your pain, which might include medications, physiotherapy and exercise, psychological therapies, relaxation and mindfulness, managing emotions related to pain, and learning pacing to avoid flare-ups.

There are so many options when it comes to accessing support for chronic pain, whether these are self-help and management techniques or more structured healthcare support such as pain clinics or management programmes. The most important thing to remember when it comes to chronic pain is that you are never alone, even if living in pain can feel isolating at times. Your loved ones and support system might never *truly* understand what it is like to live in constant pain, but they will be there to support you in your chronic pain journey in any way they can. There are also plenty of support groups and management programmes which can support you and allow you to access a community of other chronic pain patients who will understand what you're going through. As with other wellbeing concerns, try not to suffer in silence but reach out to those around you when you are ready.

Some final thoughts...

Disability can come with its own unique mental and physical challenges, whether that's learning how to pace, dealing with chronic pain, or generally looking after your wellbeing with all the challenges that get thrown your way as a disabled person. However, it's important to remember that you never have to be alone. There are many things that you can do to look after yourself and be proactive in tending to your mental and physical health. Whilst reaching out for professional help can be hard, try not to dismiss this as an option; there is no shame in asking your doctor or healthcare professional for the support that you need.

What I learned:

- Frustrating as it can be at times, pacing is key to learning to manage your fatigue when you have an energy-limiting condition.

- Remember that pacing is a very individual thing. You may have one way to pace, whilst a friend with the same diagnosis may use another. The main thing is that the way you pace is working effectively for *you*.

- Being disabled is hard and there are many challenges and curve balls that get thrown your way. It's only natural for this to have an impact on your mental health and wellbeing – we are only human, after all!

- You can try to bottle things up, but it rarely works when it comes to your mental health as things have a way of fizzing up and spilling over with time! It's much better to address your mental health and wellbeing and learn healthy coping mechanisms for when life gets hard.

- A lot of mental health and wellbeing advice sounds like common sense – sleep well, eat well, get some exercise. Although they sound basic, they do have more of an impact on your wellbeing than you might think. Try to address these basics and you will likely notice a positive impact on your overall wellbeing.

- If you are seriously struggling with your mental health, please, please, please reach out. I have been in very dark places, and it was reaching out to others that saved my life. Whether you choose to talk to a loved one, an organisation like Samaritans, or a GP, therapist, or mental health professional, things often do get better.

Reflection Time:

1. Would pacing help you to better manage your symptoms? What steps will you take to implement pacing into your daily routine?

2. Do you face any mental health difficulties due to your disability? If so, what are these difficulties?

3. From the advice in this chapter, what might help you to ease the mental health difficulties that you are experiencing? How will you incorporate these actions into your daily life?

4. Do you experience any chronic pain? How does this make you feel, physically and mentally?

5. From the advice in this chapter, what might help to alleviate your chronic pain and its physical and mental effects on you? How will you incorporate these practices into your daily life?

Chapter 9
Finding Your Freedom

Mobility aids, access, and getting around

In addition to the tips in the last chapter, there may be other practical support that can help with fatigue and pain levels, such as accessing appropriate mobility aids or asking for support to get out and about. I will always remember the day that I got my first pair of crutches, as well as the day that I received my first custom wheelchair. The first mobility aid I ever needed – back when I was able to walk a bit – was a pair of crutches. I had found the perfect pair, with comfortable moulded handles and a pattern which I'd designed myself. Unwrapping them felt like all my birthdays had come at once. I tried them and instantly knew they would transform my life, giving me greater independence and freedom.

My crutches allowed me to access the world again and walk farther and for longer without as much pain and fatigue. But I then lost the ability to walk and became a full-time wheelchair user and remain so today. I had the same feeling again when my first ever custom-made wheelchair was delivered. It was the most beautiful thing I'd ever seen with its shining chrome finish, leather trim, and bright white spokes on the wheels, just as I had designed it. It was the next step to maintaining my independence and I felt incredibly fortunate to have been able to access the exact chair that I needed with the very kind help of my parents.

Amongst the public, there is often a perception that mobility aids are something tragic, and something that disabled people must resort to using as there is something 'wrong' with us. As a disabled person, though, my mobility aids mean my freedom and independence. It took me a while to unlearn this internalised ableist view of mobility aids, but now I see them as something which bring joy, and which enable me to live the life I choose. The same can be said for being able to board accessible public transport and being able to access the places I want. When I built up the courage to use public transport with my mobility aids, it was terrifying. But at the same time, it felt like the world was opening back up to me after I had been stuck at home for so long. This chapter will look at how to get the mobility aids that you need, how to get around on public and private transport in the UK, and how to access different places as a disabled person.

Mobility Aids

Mobility aids come in all different shapes and sizes and can be used for different situations. There are walking sticks, crutches, rollators, wheelchairs and their attachments, and mobility scooters, to name but a few. One aid is not necessarily better than another; they are just suited to different tasks, and it can help to choose the best one for your specific needs. Some people – especially those with dynamic disabilities – use different aids on different days, or even within the same day depending on how their condition fluctuates. There is nothing wrong with using the aids that work best for you at different times. If using an aid will give you greater independence and mobility, it's at least worth a try!

How do you know it's time to start using a mobility aid?

A common question that comes up around all kinds of mobility aids is how you know when it's the right time to start using one, or when it's the right time to switch to a different mobility aid. Some people struggle a lot with this question, especially if they are battling internalised ableism. They might think that using a mobility aid is 'lazy' or 'giving up' or they might question whether they are 'disabled enough' to use one. Others can be confounded by the fact that the need for a mobility aid rarely happens abruptly but can instead involve more of a slow decline in your mobility. This can make it harder to know if you need a mobility aid, or if you can hold off for a little while longer without one. Deciding when it's the right time to use a mobility aid is an incredibly personal decision, and will depend on several factors including your symptoms, their severity, and your mobility.

My journey with mobility aids began with a pair of crutches. At the age of seventeen, I was experiencing severe pain in my knees, ankles, hips, and spine when I was walking. We didn't know at this point that I had Ehlers-Danlos Syndrome, but it felt excruciating

275

when I walked as my joints would often slide around in their sockets and sublux. My balance was worsening too, which had led to a series of falls and subsequent injuries. It was physiotherapist who first suggested trying a pair of crutches. I'll admit that at first, I was dubious. I was battling internalised ableism, questioning whether I was 'disabled enough' to need a mobility aid and wondering whether others would think I was 'giving up' on getting better by resorting to it. I was equally doubting whether crutches would have *that* much of an impact on my pain and fatigue. My pain was becoming so severe, though, that I was willing to try anything that might help, even in a small way.

Following my physiotherapist's advice, I did the research and settled on a well-reviewed pair of crutches with moulded handles and a funky pattern perfect for a seventeen-year-old. As soon as I slipped the cuffs over my arms and rested my weight on the crutches, I knew that this had been the right decision and that I was long overdue needing them. The pain in my spine, hips, and knees was drastically reduced, and I could walk farther and for longer with little pain with my crutches. They greatly improved my balance too, providing the stability that I needed when I began to sway. As a result, I had barely any falls when on my crutches. Although some of the internalised ableism persisted, the positive effect on my life outweighed the negative impact of some of the hurtful comments I received. Having a mobility aid that looked funky and had some of my personality injected into it helped too, as I began to feel like my crutches were simply an extension of me. My crutches revolutionised my life, giving me back the freedom and independence that I craved. My only wish is that I would have started using them sooner!

Whilst the decision to start using a mobility aid is a highly personal one, there are some things that you might want to consider if you're debating on getting one. If you experience frequent falls, pain in your legs or joints, loss of balance or dizziness, muscle weakness, vision problems affecting your mobility, difficulty with uneven surfaces, or extreme fatigue after walking short distances, these are possible signs that you might benefit from using a mobility aid. There are some other telltale signs, a few of which include:

- **Holding onto furniture.** If you hold onto furniture when you walk – maybe due to muscle weakness, fatigue, loss of balance, or difficulties with spatial awareness – you could be at risk of falls or pulling furniture over onto you. A mobility aid might be a better solution to offer you some stability as you move around your home.

- **It takes days to recover from an outing.** If pain and fatigue are making days out into a big deal, or if you must 'pay for' them by experiencing a flare-up of your symptoms for days afterwards, a mobility aid may help to alleviate some of your symptoms and make outings more comfortable for you.

- **You have frequent falls.** If you have frequent falls, it can be a sign that you might need an assistive mobility device. Some falls can cause serious injuries on top of your disability or chronic condition. Strategically placed grab rails could be a good solution here.

- **You feel forced to stay at home when the weather is bad.** When your muscle strength, vision, spatial awareness, or balance are compromised, bad weather can be daunting and dangerous. If you're feeling increasingly scared to go outside when it's wet or slippery, mobility aids might help you to regain some confidence to go outside again.

- **You decline social invitations.** For some disabled people, social invitations can be anxiety-inducing. You might feel that it's easier to stay home if you're scared of having falls, experiencing pain flares, or getting fatigued too quickly. This can have a knock-on effect on your mental health and wellbeing, leaving you feeling alone and isolated. Using a mobility aid to alleviate your symptoms can increase your comfort and confidence, allowing you to socialise with your loved ones and friends again.

- **You feel like you're losing your independence.** You might feel that you're not able to do things by yourself anymore or feel that you're relying more on others to help you to get out and about. If you are struggling with a loss of independence, trying a mobility aid could help you to tackle this and rebuild your confidence in doing things independently once more.

There are many signs that mean you might benefit from using a mobility aid, and it remains a very personal decision with many factors to consider. At the end of the day, perhaps the best piece of advice that I can give you is that, if you think that using a mobility aid might help you, the odds are that it probably will. Most importantly, you need to feel comfortable and confident about using a mobility aid, and a part of this is choosing the right aid for your needs and symptoms.

Let's look at a few different mobility aids that you could choose from, so that you can think about which might be the best fit for your circumstances. One thing to note is that, if you are in employment and need an aid to support you, Access to Work may be able to help you to fund the equipment. You can find out more about this scheme in chapter six.

Walking sticks and crutches

Walking sticks and crutches give you extra support when walking and can help you to balance better. You can borrow some types of walking sticks and crutches from the NHS by speaking to your GP, a physiotherapist, or a member of hospital staff, but you may have to pay a small deposit. There are different kinds of walking sticks and crutches, so it's crucial to find the right match for your needs. Some things to think about when selecting a stick or a crutch are:

- Making sure that they are the right height for you.

- Whether you need a stick that stands up by itself or has multiple legs.

- Whether you need the stick or crutch to be right-handed or left-handed, or whether you need a pair of them.

- Whether you need a stick or crutch with a moulded handle, or whether other types of handle would suit you better.

- Whether you need a stick with a built-in seat so you can rest.

- Whether you need a stick to go up steps.

If you are unsure which type of stick or crutch would be most appropriate for you, it's advisable to consult a professional such as your GP or a physiotherapist. They will be able to assess your needs and recommend the one that will be best suited to your needs and symptoms.

If you no longer want to use NHS sticks or want something a little more stylish, you can purchase walking sticks and crutches privately. Most basic sticks range from £5 to £30, and you can buy them from mobility shops like Ableworld or online. If you would prefer something more designer, there are some great options out there for a higher price:

- **Cool Crutches** is a UK-based and award-winning company run by a mother and daughter duo. They have a wide selection of designer sticks and crutches, including a children's range and ones with extra-wide cuffs. If nothing catches your eye, they offer a design-your-own stick or crutch service at an extra cost. Their website has useful guides on how to choose the right mobility aid for your needs, as well as a great guide to disability benefits in the UK.

- **Neo Walk** is another UK-based company which has a selection of designer walking sticks, including glittery and light-up sticks. They sell accessories too, including coloured ferrules and stick bracelets, so that you can express your personality and style. Their sticks can be made with a range of different handles to suit your needs.

- **smartCRUTCH** is a UK-based company and offers a range of coloured elbow crutches, which help to take the pressure off the wrists and hands whilst walking. They spread pressure more evenly when you are using your crutches.

- **Glamsticks** is a UK-based company and creates personalised sticks, crutches, and sight canes hand-made to your requirements. Their sticks are glittery and bedazzled with gems in all kinds of patterns and colours, if you're looking to add a bit of sparkle to your mobility aid.

Walking sticks and crutches can be a fantastic option if you're looking for an aid that will reduce pressure and pain on your joints, help with your balance, and build your confidence to get out and about again. There are plenty of ways to personalise your aids or to purchase one which reflects your personality to give you even more of a confidence boost.

Walking Frames

A walking frame – also known as a Zimmer frame, a walker, or a rollator – is a mobility aid which offers support and stability if you have difficulty walking and balancing. You can borrow a walking frame from the NHS if you speak to your GP or physiotherapist; as with sticks and crutches, you may have to pay a small deposit. There are different kinds of walking frame, so there are some factors that you might wish to take into consideration when selecting one to try:

- Make sure that it's the correct height for you to ensure you are comfortable using it.

- Whether you want to only use it indoors, as frames without wheels are best for this.

- Whether you're strong enough to lift a frame without wheels.

- Whether you want to get out and about outdoors, as frames with wheels are best for this.

- Whether you need a seat, basket, or tray attached.

- Whether you need to fold it to get it in and out of a car.

If you are unsure which type of walking frame would be most appropriate for you, it's advisable to consult a professional such as your GP or a physiotherapist.

Alternatively, you can privately purchase walking frames and rollators. A standard walking frame can roughly cost between £30 and £50, either from a specialist mobility store or on the internet.

There are plenty of ways you can customise them on a budget too, including coloured or patterned tapes, spray paints, stickers, or vinyl. If you would prefer something more designer, there are some great options out there:

- **ByAcre** is advertised as the lightest rollator in the world. They offer various stylish, functional, and modern rollators with wheels for indoor and outdoor use. Some of their rollators are foldable to easily transport them in a car and come with a seat built-in to allow you to rest. They have options with baskets too if you need to transport things with your rollator.

- **Rollz Motion and Rollz Electric** are rollators which come in various designs and configurations. Some styles can transform into a transit wheelchair and even an electric transit wheelchair for high pain and fatigue days. Rollz offers accessories for your rollator too, such as umbrellas, trays, lights, walking stick holders, back support, and travel covers.

Walkers are a good option if you sometimes need more stability than a stick or crutch can offer, or if you need to be able to easily sit down or carry things whilst you're moving about.

Sight Canes

Sight canes – sometimes known as 'white canes' or 'guide canes' – are mobility aids used by blind and partially sighted people to navigate the world safely by providing tactile feedback about the environment around them. You can often get sight canes through the

NHS, either by borrowing them or having them provided after a needs assessment by a low-vision clinic. Under the Care Act 2014, local authorities should provide you with aids and minor adaptations up to the value of £1,000. If you need a sight cane to support your independence, it's worth speaking to your local council to see what they can provide you with. This includes sight canes but may cover other aids or adaptations that will support you, such as products that help in the kitchen or when bathing. If you need advice on the right cane for you, or to arrange cane training, you can contact your local authority's sensory team or orientation specialist to get assessed for a cane and learn how to use it safely.

When considering which sight cane is the best fit for you, there are a few things you might want to consider. In the UK, a white cane signifies that the user is blind, whilst a white cane with red stripes indicates a dual disability, such as vision and hearing loss, or someone who is deafblind. There are also different kinds of tips available for your cane which have different uses and benefits. A few of these tips include:

- **Roller 'marshmallow' tip.** This tip rolls over the ground through a constant contact technique. Made from durable material, it can be longer lasting than other tips.

- **Rolling ball tip.** A larger ball that rolls over the ground with a constant contact technique. It is designed to reduce catching on small cracks and bumps in the pavement.

- **Jumbo roller tip.** This tip is shaped like a disc and rolls from side to side using a constant contact technique. Its design helps to avoid snagging on cracks in the pavement, and it is made from a durable, long-lasting material.

- **Pencil tip.** A straight tip with a rounded point at the end, this is designed to be used by tapping on the ground in a two- or three-point touch cane technique.

- **Omni-sense tip**. Made from a combination of plastic wheels and rollers, the tip is designed to move in all directions with 360-degree motion using the constant contact technique. Its design helps it to move easily over uneven surfaces.

If you are unsure which type of cane and tip are right for you, work with the sensory team from your local authority. They can assess your needs and provide the appropriate mobility training you need to complete before becoming a sight cane user.

If you want a more bespoke cane, you can purchase them privately. The **Royal National Institute of Blind People (RNIB)** has an online shop where you can purchase different colour sight canes, including children's canes, for around £30 to £90. If you're looking for something a bit more high-tech, **WeWalk** has a smart sight cane with a range of features for around £700, although you can get cheaper refurbished ones. The smart cane has enhanced obstacle detection, an intelligent voice assistant, connection to your phone via Bluetooth, accessible navigation instructions, live public transport information, and voice feedback to help you explore the world around you. Another option is **Glamsticks,** a UK-based company which creates personalised sight canes hand-made to your requirements from around £120. Their sticks are often glittery or bedazzled with gems, if you're looking to add a bit of sparkle to your cane.

Mobility Scooters

Mobility scooters can be useful if you are struggling to walk long distances due to pain, fatigue, or mobility issues, provided that you are able to easily get on and off the scooter. Unfortunately, mobility scooters are not typically available on the NHS, but you can purchase them privately. Depending on the make, model, and specification, mobility scooters tend to cost between £500 and £5000. If you are struggling with the cost, Better Mobility has a list of charities that can help pay towards the cost of the scooter. You could also try fundraising independently, such as on JustGiving. If you receive the higher mobility component of PIP, you can either hire or buy a mobility scooter through the Motability Scheme;[45] this allows some people to use their benefits to pay for a mobility scooter. If you only need a scooter for big days out, many attractions

---

[45] Please note that all information was correct at time of publication [31 October 2025]. Please always check Government websites for the most up-to-date information in cases of changes to this scheme.

such as zoos, theme parks, gardens, and so forth have mobility scooters that you can hire on long days out for a small fee or deposit.

It is recommended that you try different types of mobility scooters before you select one to buy, to ensure that your chosen one meets your mobility needs. There are various types of scooters, including pavement scooters, road-legal scooters, folding scooters, and car-boot scooters. When trying different models out, there are some questions that you might want to ask yourself to help you choose the best one for your needs:

- How often do you need to use the scooter?

- What do you need it for? For example, roads, pavements, off-road?

- Do you need your mobility scooter to fit into a car?

- Where will you store your scooter at home?

- How easy and how costly it is to maintain and repair? Can you easily get parts and specialist engineers for it?

- How will you steer the scooter? Some have special levers to make them easier to steer if you have joint problems or arthritis in your hands.

- Can you safely get on and off the scooter?

Mobility scooters offer an alternative to walking long distances and can help those with disabilities or mobility issues to regain their independence. They can enable you to travel farther, with less pain and fatigue, and participate more fully in daily activities and social events.

Manual and Electric Wheelchairs

Wheelchairs are another option for those who cannot walk at all or who struggle with walking, and who may find it difficult to transfer on or off a mobility scooter. There are many different types of wheelchairs, including manual transit or self-propel active chairs, as well as a range of electric wheelchairs. Just as there are various types of wheelchairs, there are several ways to acquire one depending on your individual circumstances.

One way to acquire a wheelchair is through the **NHS wheelchair services** in your area, to which your GP, physiotherapist, or member of hospital staff can refer you. In some parts of the UK, you may even be able to self-refer to wheelchair services without seeing your GP. Your local wheelchair services will then carry out an assessment and decide if you need a wheelchair and, if so, what type. If you would prefer a different chair to the one offered, you may be able to get a voucher or a personal wheelchair budget instead, which allows you to pay towards the cost of a different wheelchair.[46]

---

[46] Please note that all information was correct at time of publication [31 October 2025]. Please always check NHS websites or with your GP for the most up-to-date information in cases of changes to this scheme.

Alternatively, if you are in work and need a manual or electric wheelchair to help with your job, you may be able to apply for **Access to Work** support to help towards the cost. Your Access to Work grant can be combined with your personal wheelchair budget to increase the funding available to you. Another option is the **Motability scheme**, who can help if you want to hire or purchase an electric wheelchair, if you receive the higher mobility rate of PIP. If you would like to find out more about the Motability scheme, continue reading later in this chapter.

If you do not need a wheelchair for long-term use and don't want to invest in the cost of one, there are other options available to you. If you need support after an injury or operation, you might be able to borrow an **NHS** wheelchair for a short period of time. You can ask your GP, physiotherapist, or hospital specialist about this option. If you need a wheelchair when you are out and about, **Shopmobility** lends wheelchairs and powered scooters to people who are disabled so that they can shop or visit leisure facilities in their town or city centre. Hire costs can vary depending on your location but are typically very low cost or even free.

For many, a wheelchair is a big investment and so you want to make the right choice. It's often worth trying different makes and model of wheelchairs to find the best fit for your needs. There are some things you may wish to consider when it comes to selecting the right chair:

- Will you push it yourself or do you want to be pushed by someone else, or a mixture of the two?

- How often do you need to use your wheelchair?

- Do you need to use it indoors or outdoors, or both?

- Do you need a chair that can fold or dismantle to be put in a car or other small spaces, such as for storage?

- Do you need to be able to lift a chair across your body if you are driving a car? Or will you store your wheelchair in your car another way, such as by using a car hoist?

- Can the wheelchair fit around your house and are the doors wide enough to accommodate it?

- How comfortable is the chair for you, especially if you will be sat in it for long periods?

- How easy and how costly is the wheelchair to repair and maintain?

These questions can help you to narrow down the type of wheelchair you need, so that you can focus your search and try out ones which meet your specifications. When I first became a wheelchair user, though, I had absolutely no idea which makes and models of wheelchair were out there and which might suit my needs. There are so many options out there that it can sometimes feel confusing of where to start. Here are some makes of wheelchair that might help you to begin your search:

-   **The Excel G-Explorer** – this is a good starter chair for the price. It can manage most terrains and the weight of the chair is not too considerable.

-   **Quickie**

-   **RGK**

-   **TiLite**

-   **Kuschall**

-   **Permobil**

-   **Omeo**

-   **Whill mobility scooters**, from TGA Mobility

These are just a few of the wheelchair makers available in the UK. When it comes to selecting your wheelchair, my main advice would be to try as many different models as you can. It's then worth comparing them and weighing up the pros and cons of each to decide on the chair that best suits your needs. Although there can be stigma attached to them, wheelchairs can give you so much freedom and independence, so it's worth investing in the one that suits your needs to offer you the best support.

Power Attachments

Whilst wheelchairs can be incredible, sometimes it's nice to have a bit of an extra helping hand when you're self-propelling and your arms and shoulders are aching! This can come in the form of power attachments, sometimes called power add-ons or power assists. These are devices which can be attached to manual wheelchairs to quickly and easily turn them into powered chairs. They're perfect for if you need that little bit of extra support – whether for pain, fatigue, or other symptoms – and to make your manual wheelchair perform even better for your needs. Power-assist devices also reduce wear and tear on your joints by taking the strain and can be great for those with energy-limiting conditions. They are therefore ideal for active users, as they can increase the distance you can travel over tougher terrains and give an extra power boost to your chair, helping with many of the symptoms which can come with using a wheelchair.

There are lots of different powered add-ons on the market, including pull- and push-devices. It can sometimes feel rather confusing to look at a range of products and know which ones to select to best suit your needs. To help with this, here are a few questions which you might want to consider:

- How do you want the device to attach to your wheelchair? Push-devices typically attach underneath or at the back of the chair, whilst pull devices tend to go on the front instead.

- How often do you intend to use your power attachment device?

- Do you need a device which is quite compact for limited storage space, or could you accommodate a larger device that does not compact down very much?

- Do you need to be able to lift the power attachment into your car? Is your car big enough and are you able to lift a potentially heavy piece of equipment? Or would you need a car hoist to help you get it into the car?

Purchasing a power attachment is a big investment – just like the wheelchair itself – so quite a few people find it hard to make this big decision. My advice would be to take your time and to try out a range of attachments before you settle on the one which best suits your needs. Below is a list of some of the most common power assist devices on the market at the moment, to help you to get started in your search:

- **Permobil Smart Drive MX2+.** The Smart Drive is a light-weight power assist device for manual wheelchairs. It mainly helps with areas where it's hard to push, such as going up ramps, on the pavement, on thick carpet, and travelling long distances. It's very compact and discrete, attaching to the bar underneath your wheelchair, and has great manoeuvrability. It can be operated either by buttons or by the Push Tracker wristband, which senses your movements to control the Smart Drive.

- **SMOOV.** The SMOOV is an electric assist device that you can easily attach or detach from your wheelchair when you need a little extra power. This unit can significantly improve your mobility, with a range of up to 12 miles and a speed of up to 6mph.

- **Streetjet.** The Streetjet is a high-performance pull device capable of tackling tough terrain and reaching distances of up to

50km. It is quick and easy to connect to your wheelchair using a patented clamp system, meaning that – unlike other competitor models – you do not need any components to remain on your wheelchair to attach the device. The Streetjet also has a wheel stand, which helps to keep it in an upright position and to roll it easily towards your chair for docking.

- **Empulse F35.** At 7.5kg, the Empulse F35 is marketed as the lightest and smallest manual wheelchair pull device currently available. It offers a great balance between size and practicality, with a range of up to 15km and a speed of up to 15kph.

- **Triride.** Triride offers electric pull devices capable of providing manual wheelchair users with amazing mobility in both day-to-day life and leisure time. There are a wide range of Triride models to meet your needs, whether that's following city routes, cycle lanes, roads, or mountain paths.

- **Alber E-Motion wheels.** The E-motion wheels are activated via the push rims and are designed to take the strain off manual wheelchair users. Integrated into the wheel hubs, the electric motors allow the wheelchair user to put much less effort into travelling greater distances, on different terrains or slopes. Every pulse on the push rims is registered by a sensor and translated into the right amount of electrical assistance.

- **Empulse Wheeldrive power-assisted wheels.** WheelDrive provides extra pushing power when self-propelling and allows you to continuously drive due to the unique double rim system. The wheels are easy to program according to your needs, and reduce strain on your muscles and joints, allowing you to stay active and independent.

These are just a few of the power-assist options available in the UK currently. Power assist devices are not for everyone but can help to protect the longevity of your joints and your independence as a wheelchair user, especially as they reduce the strain on your muscles and joints. Whether you're looking for a pull-device or a push-device, there are plenty of options available out there and, if you're not sure, head out and try some to see what you think!

Assistance Dogs

Whilst perhaps not typically what comes to mind when you think about mobility aids, assistance dogs help with their handler's mobility and independence. In the UK, assistance dogs are defined under the Equality Act 2010 as dogs trained to support disabled people with disabilities affecting their sight, hearing, mobility, and other issues, or trained by certain Assistance Dog UK (ADUK) charities to assist a disabled person with prescribed tasks. Under the Equality Act 2010, it is also unlawful to discriminate against assistance dog users and fully trained assistance dogs have full rights of access to public spaces and services.

Assistance Dogs UK (ADUK) is a coalition of organisations which train assistance dogs and which have been accredited by Assistance Dogs International (ADI) or the International Guide Dog

Federation (IGDF). ADUK members are generally non-profit organisations and work to the highest standards of dog training and welfare. The ADUK member organisations are currently as follows:

- **Autism Dogs.** Autism Dogs train dogs for both adults and children with autism.

- **Bravehound.** Bravehound is a Scottish charity which trains assistance dogs for veterans with a diagnosed mental health condition, such as Post Traumatic Stress Disorder (PTSD).

- **Canine Partners.** Canine Partners offers various services for people with physical disabilities, including fully trained assistance dogs, home assistance canines, and canine companions who provide emotional support and companionship to disabled adults and children.

- **Darwin Dogs.** Darwin Dogs partners with disabled people to help train them to handle their own dogs as assistance dogs for diagnosed mental health conditions or people with autism.

- **Dog A.I.D.** Dog A.I.D supports disabled people to train their own pet dogs as assistance dogs.

- **Dogs for Autism.** Dogs for Autism trains assistance dogs for people with a diagnosis of autism.

- **Dogs for Good.** Dogs for Good provide assistance dogs for families with an autistic child and for physically disabled adults and children. They also have community dogs, providing animal-assisted activities and treatments for diverse needs.

- **Guide Dogs.** Guide Dogs offers guide dogs for adults and young people who are either blind or partially sighted and who need support with mobility and independent travel. They further provide buddy dogs to offer emotional support and companionship for children who are blind or partially sighted.

- **Hearing Dogs.** Hearing Dogs offers hearing dogs and sound support dogs for children and adults with a hearing impairment. Alternatively, they provide Confidence and Companion Dogs for people with hearing impairments.

- **Medical Detection Dogs.** Medical Detection Dogs provides dogs which can medically alert as they have been trained to recognise the odour of various conditions and diseases.

- **Service Dogs UK.** Service Dogs UK offers trauma support dogs and assistance dogs to help members of the Armed Forces and Emergency Services who have served and who have PTSD.

- **Support Dogs.** Support Dogs provide assistance dogs for children with autism and epilepsy seizure alert dogs for adults over the age of 16. They further support people with physical disabilities to train their own pet dogs to be assistance dogs.

- **The Seeing Dogs Alliance.** The Seeing Dogs Alliance offers fully trained guide dogs to support adults who are blind or partially sighted.

- **Veterans with Dogs.** Veterans with Dogs offer assistance dogs for ex-service and military personnel who are diagnosed with a mental health condition.

297

All ADUK members and candidate organisations use positive reinforcement training – sometimes known as reward-based training – to train their dogs. If you are considering applying for an assistance dog, it can help to speak with a couple of charities that offer dogs that would meet your needs. They will have different criteria and requirements to apply for a dog, so it is worth researching and finding a charity that fits with what you are looking for and the tasks you need a dog to assist you with.

There are benefits to acquiring an assistance dog through a charitable organisation, whether they are ADUK certified or not. Non-profit organisations often provide dogs either for free or for minimal cost, and you can be assured that dogs are trained to the highest public access standards. But they do have eligibility criteria and requirements for you to qualify for a dog and can tend to have quite long waitlists; in some cases, you may have to wait a couple of years after being approved to eventually be partnered with your dog.

If a non-profit organisation is not the route for you, there are other options available to acquire an assistance dog. In the UK, there is no legal requirement to have your dog trained by a specific organisation or charity, meaning that you can instead self-train an assistance dog if you wish. Many people who choose this route find it helpful to get the support of professional trainers or other organisations, such as **Adolescent Dogs**, who offer programmes specifically for owner-trained assistance dogs. Other organisations, such as **WKD Dogs**, offer fully trained assistance dogs for purchase or you can provide a dog, and they will train it to your needs for a fee. To be an assistance dog, your dog will need to have a high level of obedience and specialised skills. Whilst public access tests are not mandatory in the UK, many owners still choose to undergo them to ensure that their dog meets the required standard.

Self-training an assistance dog can be beneficial if you do not meet the eligibility criteria or requirements for ADUK or other charities. It equally offers you a greater degree of control over how you train your dog and the kinds of tasks you train them to do, offering a more bespoke training option. Wait times for self-trained assistance dogs can be much shorter than waiting for a non-profit to provide a dog. However, self-training an assistance dog is a demanding process and support from professional trainers or organisations is recommended. Either purchasing a fully trained assistance dog or paying a professional to help you to train your own dog can be pricey. You will also need to ensure that your pet insurance covers public liability if you plan to train your dog for public access.

Whether you apply to a non-profit organisation or self-train your own dog, assistance dogs can be an incredible support to their handlers, enabling them to reclaim their freedom, confidence, and independence. Many assistance dog handlers greatly value the companionship, the close bond they develop with their canine companion, and the emotional benefits that come with raising a dog too. If you enjoy working with animals and can identify ways that a dog could help you to improve your mobility and independence, then it might be worth looking into whether an assistance dog could support you.

Some final reflections on mobility aids...

Mobility aids are integral to helping disabled people to get out and about and in regaining their confidence and independence. Whilst stigma unfortunately persists around the use of mobility aids among the public, this is not how most disabled people perceive their aids. They instead associate their aids with increased joy and freedom. Mobility aids are only one factor in increasing our mobility and independence, though. There are many transport systems in the UK which offer services and accommodations for disabled people, and which help them to mobilise around the world. Let's look at our rights on public transport, and the transport options that are available to disabled people, in greater depth.

Your rights on public transport

Under the Equality Act 2010, public transport in the UK must be accessible to disabled people and service providers are legally required to make reasonable adjustments. This might include accepting assistance dogs or providing priority seating for people with disabilities. It might also cover having wide doors and designated spaces for wheelchairs, or fitting ramps on some buses, trains, and trams. It would be a reasonable adjustment to provide free tickets for carers or personal assistants, as well as requiring drivers or conductors to provide reasonable assistance to disabled passengers. Whilst all public transport providers must offer an accessible service, it's still a good idea to book support in advance if you can, especially if you are travelling from a smaller station or bus or tram stop.

The Department for Transport set out its priorities for improving disabled access in the 2018 Inclusive Transport Strategy (ITS). This included the promotion of passenger rights, better staff training, and improved information across all modes of transport. Part 12 of the Equality Act 2010 contains provision specific to trains, buses, coaches, taxis, and private hire vehicles. This means that public transport services cannot discriminate against a disabled person, and services need to make reasonable adjustments to enable disabled people to use their service independently.

Now that we better understand our rights on public and private transport, let's take the time to look at each mode of transport to see how it can be made accessible and how you can access this more independently.

Train travel and the London Underground

Trains generally tend to be quite an accessible mode of transport, if the right support is put in place for you. All main train operators and stations are required to create and comply with an Accessible

Travel Plan (ATP). This should include what services and facilities are available and how you can get assistance. You can request a copy of the ATP from the train operator. The Office of Rail and Road is the body which holds your train operator to account on their ATP and they can review an operator's policy if they believe that it is not being followed.

Mainline trains must have a mandatory number of spaces for wheelchair users and there must be an accessible toilet next to each. Just remember to put your brakes on or switch your power off when using the wheelchair space to keep you safe! There are no mandatory requirements about mobility scooters, though, so it's best to check the operator's ATP. Whilst trains in the UK are not legally required to have audio induction loops – or T-loops – most do, and all stations are required to have them too. Some stations have braille and audio maps to help blind and partially sighted people with navigation. Station employees and train personnel are required to make reasonable adjustments to help passengers, including assistance with boarding, navigating stations, purchasing tickets, finding seats, and receiving information. Most stations have Assisted Travel Lounges where you can go for assistance, and some lounges even have sensory spaces. Network Rail has also committed to making all their managed stations autism-friendly by the end of 2025.

Whilst these adjustments are intended to help you to navigate trains independently, you can alternatively give National Rail train companies advance notice if you think you'll need any help from staff during your journey. You can do this via the Passenger Assistance app or their booking website. The app and website have been designed in consultation with disabled people and are suitable for screen readers. You can set up your profile by adding information about yourself, such as whether you're a wheelchair user, whether you have an assistance dog, whether you have a non-apparent condition you need support with, whether you have a mental health or neurodivergent condition, or whether you have any sensory disabilities or needs. After setting up your profile, you can let Passenger Assistance know the details of your journey and the types of support you will need. Your request will then be sent directly to the train operator, who will organise the assistance for you, and you will get a confirmation notice once this is sorted. If you are unable to plan ahead, you can instead turn up at any station without a booking and ask them for assistance with access. If you're at all unhappy with the service you get, you can complain to the train operator directly. If they cannot resolve the complaint, you may be able to complain to the Rail Ombudsman if the train company has joined the scheme.

As a disabled person, you may be eligible for discounts on your rail travel. You might be able to get a Disabled Person's Railcard that gives you a third off rail travel for you and an adult companion. You must provide evidence of a relevant disability, and you can find out further information about whether you're eligible on the railcard website. If you are blind or partially sighted and travelling with a companion, you can get a discount on rail travel without having a disabled person's railcard. More information can be found on the National Rail website.

On the London Underground – also known at the Tube – Transport for London (TfL) use a service called 'turn-up-and-go' (TUAG) to help disabled people with access to stations and services. You do not need to pre-book assistance but can simply turn up and ask a member of staff to help you to board the train or meet you at your destination. TfL offer a travel support card that you can order online or download and print and home if you need help with communicating your access needs and information. It can be used on any TfL service. The TfL website has a step-free Tube map, as well as a page called 'How to Plan an Accessible Journey'. You can contact TfL Accessibility in the first instance if you wish to make a complaint about your journey or the access that was available. If assistance has not been provided, then TfL will usually offer you a full refund for your journey.

There are some great access options and discounts available if you are a disabled person travelling via train. Having travelled by train many times, my best advice would be to book assistance in advance, if you can. It helps the train operators to prepare ahead, and it gives you confirmation that your assistance will be ready for you at the station. It can be a good idea to check in with a member of station staff once you arrive, so that they know they need to support you. Most station staff are friendly and more than happy to help, but if you are not happy with the assistance that you receive, it's worth highlighting this to someone so they can improve their service for other disabled travellers.

Bus, coach, and tram travel

There are regulations which set out how accessible your local buses and coaches should be, which are known as the Public Service Vehicles Accessibility Regulations (PSVAR). It states that on buses and coaches, there should be lifts or ramps to enable wheelchair users to board, there must be slip-resistant flooring, and both external and internal steps must conform to the PSVAR requirements, such as being covered in slip-resistant material and being highlighted by high-contrast reflective tape. There must be route and destination displays on the outside of the vehicle and colour-contrasting handrails. The PSVAR requires that there is enough space under or next to at least one priority seat to comfortably accommodate an assistance dog, although there is no limit to the number of assistance dogs that can be on one vehicle.

The law states that bus and coach drivers must give reasonable assistance to disabled people, such as helping them to get on and off the bus. But this does not mean physically lifting passengers or heavy mobility equipment. Instead, it could include getting out a ramp to allow a wheelchair or mobility aid user to get on or off the bus. Bus drivers should ensure that you can access the wheelchair space if it is available and make sure that you are safely positioned before the vehicle moves. Wheelchair users should be given priority over items like luggage or pushchairs; if there is an item in the wheelchair space when you try to board the bus, the driver should ask the owner to move this but if they refuse, the driver cannot force them to do so. There is no requirement for bus operators to allow disabled passengers to travel with a mobility scooter. Those that need a scooter may need to obtain a permit to present to the bus driver.

You can get a disabled person's bus pass from your local Council for free bus and tram travel in England. It's only valid at certain times, such as 9:30am to 11pm on most days, or anytime on a Saturday, Sunday, or bank holiday. You can find out if you are eligible and apply via the government website. Buses, coaches, and trams can be great ways to travel as a disabled person, as they have various accommodations, making them a generally quite accessible mode of transport for a range of disabilities.

Car travel, Blue Badges, and the Motability Scheme

Cars can be a fantastic way to travel and offer more flexibility and independence than public transport. There are many adaptations that can be fitted to your car to enable you to drive safely with various disabilities. Adaptations can include push/pull accelerator and brake hand controls, steering aids, hoists, swivel seats, transfer plates, wheelchair or boot hoists, electronic accelerators, or entirely wheelchair accessible vehicles. You can request assessments at

306

driving centres for the disabled to test different adaptations and figure out which ones will allow you to drive safely and independently.

Whilst many disabled people can drive, you must tell the DVLA if you develop a 'notifiable' medical condition or disability, or if your condition gets worse after you receive your licence. A 'notifiable' condition includes anything that could affect your ability to drive safely, such as diabetes or taking insulin, blindness or becoming partially sighted, syncope, heart conditions, sleep apnoea, epilepsy and seizures, strokes, or glaucoma. You must surrender your licence to the DVLA if any of the following are true:

- Your doctor tells you to stop driving for 3 months or more.

- Your medical condition(s) affect(s) your ability to drive safely and lasts for 3 months or more.

- You do not meet the required standards for driving because of your medical condition.

Driving a car is one thing, but many disabled people also need accessible parking close to their location to enable them to access places independently via car. The Blue Badge Scheme helps people with mobility difficulties or disabilities to park closer to their desired location.[47] You can apply for a Blue Badge for yourself, or on behalf

---

[47] Please note that all information was correct at time of publication [31 October 2025]. Please always check Government or local council websites for the most up-to-date information in cases of changes to this scheme.

of someone else, or for an organisation that transports people with disabilities. Some people automatically qualify for a Blue Badge, and you can find out if you meet these eligibility criteria on the government website. You might still be able to qualify for a Blue Badge if you have mobility difficulties, find walking challenging, have a life-limiting illness, have a child with a medical condition, have severe anxiety, or have difficulty planning and following a journey. Your local council will decide whether you are eligible for a badge, and they cannot start the application process until they have all the relevant evidence and information. Blue Badges are intended for on-street parking only. Off-street parking – such as that offered by hospitals, supermarkets, or shopping centres – are covered by different rules, although many do still offer disabled parking bays for which you need a Blue Badge. If you are unsure whether you are eligible for a badge, it is often worth putting in an application anyway to let your Council decide whether you qualify – you've nothing to lose and everything to gain!

Another scheme which facilitates car travel for disabled people is the Motability Scheme.[48] The scheme allows you to use your benefits to lease a brand-new car or wheelchair-accessible vehicle (WAV). It covers your insurance, your breakdown cover, and servicing too and supports charging the vehicle if you choose an

---

[48] Please note that all information was correct at time of publication [31 October 2025]. Please always check Government websites for the most up-to-date information in cases of changes to this scheme.

electric model. If you do not need a car, you can instead use your benefits to lease a mobility scooter or electric wheelchair under the Motability Scheme. You can read more about this option earlier in this chapter. Different vehicles suit different people, and there is a wide selection of vehicles available on the Motability Scheme. If you visit a dealership that supports the scheme, they can assist you in making the right choice for you and your needs. It's important to note that you can still get a Motability vehicle even if you are not the driver or cannot drive; for instance, if you are blind and receive the higher mobility component of PIP, you can still order a car but name someone else as the designated driver.

You can start applying online if you want a car or a WAV under the Motability Scheme. Once you've chosen the vehicle for you, visit the Motability Scheme dealer and they will finish your application and order the vehicle for you. Once your vehicle arrives, the Motability Scheme then receives your monthly mobility payments straight from your benefits provider to make payment simple. Depending on the vehicle you choose, you may need to pay an advance payment to order the vehicle. Full information about each vehicle and any advance payment you would need to cover can be found on the Motability website. If you would struggle to cover the advance payment and the cost of any adaptations you need, you can apply to the Motability Foundation for financial help. Finally, once your vehicle is ready, you can either pick it up from your local car dealership, or if it is a WAV, it may be delivered straight to your home.

A final useful tip for driving as a disabled person, especially if you are a wheelchair user or have mobility issues, is to download the **FuelService app.** This can help if filling up your car with fuel is challenging due to your disability. It is a free app available on Android and iOS and is designed to help disabled drivers find assistance with refuelling their vehicle. It shows the user which nearby petrol stations participate in the scheme. Once you choose a petrol station, the app will connect you with your selected station to ensure that help is available when you arrive. The app will alert the attendant to your arrival, so that they can come and refuel your car and help with payment, making refuelling an easier and more accessible process.

Driving or travelling via car can often be the quickest and one of the most accessible ways for you to travel locally, especially if you can access a car with the right adaptations for you. Both the Blue Badge Scheme and the Motability Scheme are amazing ventures to make car travel more accessible for those with disabilities by enabling them to regain their independence. My advice would be to apply to both schemes if you are eligible, as there are so many benefits to both, even if you are a passenger princess like me!

Air travel

Airlines and airports all have various facilities for people with different disabilities. It is advisable to check out in advance whether your local airport has the facilities and support that you need. It is also a good idea to tell your airline at least 48 hours in advance if you need support, and what kind of support you need.

If you have a sensory, physical, or learning disability, you can access support at airports and certain support on the plane. At the airport, you can request help at specific arrival points, such as terminal entrances or transport exchanges. You can further ask for help to reach check-in, help with registration, help to move through the airport, or support to board the plane. For most airlines, you can travel with up to two items of mobility equipment free of charge; this will not count as part of your baggage allowance. Often, though, you cannot take your own wheelchair into the passenger cabin of the plane, as it will need to be stored in the hold instead. It's a good idea to speak to your airline to find out what help is available for you when you are boarding and tell them as soon as possible if you will be taking a battery-powered wheelchair or mobility aid, as only certain batteries are flight-safe. When on the plane, you can ask attendants to give you information about the flight in a way that you understand, as well as help moving about the plane, and finding a seat that is suited to your needs. If you are not self-reliant, it's often a good idea to travel with a companion who can help you with feeding, breathing, taking medication, or using the toilet.

Flying can be quite an anxiety-inducing experience when you have a disability, as there are lots of additional factors to consider. However, by planning ahead and communicating clearly with your airline or travel provider about your needs, you can get a clear steer on what support is available for you and what to expect when flying with a disability.

Taxis, Ubers, and other private hire vehicles

Taxis and private hire vehicles such as Ubers can be a good way to travel and give you independence if you're disabled, especially for those who cannot drive. I often hop in Ubers as an active wheelchair user, as it's a handy way to get around and you can request assistance via the app.

In the UK, it's against the law for drivers of taxis and private hire vehicles to refuse to book a vehicle or take you on a journey because you are disabled or because you have an assistance dog. Drivers and operators must give you reasonable assistance to use their service, and they cannot charge you extra for this. Drivers may be exempt from giving physical help, though, if they themselves have a disability or medical condition. If not, the help that drivers ought to provide includes help finding the vehicle, help getting in and out, help stowing a mobility aid, help reading out the total on the taximeter, and help explaining which route they're taking.

In larger cities across the UK, licensed taxis must be wheelchair accessible. To find out if there are any near you, you can contact the taxi licensing office at your local council, as they will have a list of accessible vehicles in your area. Not all private hire vehicles like Ubers must be wheelchair accessible, though. If you need a wheelchair accessible vehicle, it's often a good idea to request this in advance of your journey to ensure availability. There are some specialist private hire firms across the UK who offer accessible and wheelchair-adapted services. It can be worth researching local services in your area to find the best fit for your needs.

Ferry and boat travel

Ferries and boats can be an alternative and accessible way to travel to get abroad, and there are often adjustments in place for disabled people. Rights of disabled maritime passengers are set out in retained EU law. This means that disabled passengers have the right to travel by boat at the same price as any other non-disabled passenger, and to bring wheelchairs, mobility equipment, or assistance dogs as required.

Many ferries are accessible to travellers with various disabilities and wheelchair users. It's advisable to contact your ferry operator at least 48 hours before you travel to let them know what kind of support or assistance you will need. It's also important that you familiarise yourself with the layout of the ship, as its design can make it difficult for some disabled passengers to negotiate independently. If possible, it can be helpful to travel with an able-bodied companion to assist you during your journey. Different ships tend to have different mobility support and assistive features, so it is best to consult with your ferry operator as early as possible to discuss the support available on the ship you'll be sailing on. Travelling by ferry or boat as a disabled person may seem daunting at first, but with pre-planning and clear communication with your ferry operator, you can ensure that you are prepared and confident for your journey.

Travelling with an assistance dog

If you want to travel with an assistance dog, there are certain things that it can be helpful for you to consider in advance of your journey. Whatever mode of transport you're using, it's best if the dog wears its harness or identification jacket and that you always have its ID tag and other documentation with you. Alternatively, you might want to consider whether it's appropriate to take your assistance dog on your journey with you. If you are unsure, it can help to contact the charity or organisation who trained your dog for further advice or consult your trainer or veterinarian if your dog is owner-trained. It's often a good idea to get a veterinary examination for your dog prior to travel to ensure that they are healthy enough for the journey. You might want to think about possible veterinary care whilst you are away, too, as well as any language barriers and obtaining suitable insurance. You and your veterinarian should always consider whether your travels might cause stress for your dog, such as:

314

- Working your dog in a new and unfamiliar environment.

- Potentially working your dog in a less accessible environment than you're both used to.

- Working your dog in a different climate.

- Breaking your dog's normal routine.

- Staying in accommodation that is not your dog's home environment.

If you are concerned that travelling with your dog might cause undue stress, it is worth speaking with the organisation who trained your dog, your trainer, or your veterinarian and seek advice on any steps that you can take to prepare your dog and reduce their stress.

Different modes of transport offer different levels of support for disabled passengers travelling with assistance dogs. When travelling by air, you should ideally inform your airline or tour operator that you intend to fly with your assistance dog at least 48 hours before departure so that they can make suitable arrangements to support you. Airlines can ask for evidence that your assistance dog has been trained by a recognised organisation, such as those listed on Assistance Dogs International (ADI). You will need to check with your airline or booking agent whether ID is required and what ID you will need for owner-trained dogs.

It can further help to contact the airport directly to ensure that everything is in place to support you and your dog on the day of travel. At the airport, you should be offered the opportunity to spend your dog before passing through security and departures. You and your dog will often be boarded onto the aircraft first, as recognised assistance dogs can travel with their handlers in the aircraft cabin. Your dog may be provided with floor space in the seat next to you or they may ask your dog to lie across your feet. Depending on your journey and the travel time, it is worth considering both options and which airline(s) offer the best solution for you and your dog. You might want to think about water for your dog, as liquids are often restricted in airport security departments, although you can usually buy water once you have passed through security.

When travelling by car, there are a couple of options for your dog. If they must travel with you in the front footwell, do not disengage the passenger airbag and ensure that your dog is always lying down. If there is space, it can help to move the passenger seat forwards and place your dog in the footwell behind, supervised by a person sat behind the driver. For longer journeys, you'll need to make sure that your dog is secure in the vehicle. This can either be in the boot behind the back seats with a dog guard, or secure on the back seats with a car harness. It's advisable that your dog is wearing a collar with an ID tag during your journey.

For long journeys, you must give your dog frequent rest stops. At pet stores and online, you can purchase a range of travel equipment for dogs including travel bowls and water bottles. If you can, it's often recommended to avoid feeding your dog immediately before travelling and to ideally allow at least two hours between a meal and a journey. You might want to have a clean-up kit in case your dog becomes ill in the back of the vehicle. If you need to feed your dog on the journey, try and do this on a rest break and give plenty of time for your dog to spend. You could instead leave feeding your dog until you have reached your destination. Make sure that your vehicle has adequate ventilation for your dog, and that you avoid leaving your car in direct sunlight or temperature extremes. Do not leave your dog unattended in the car and take them with you if possible.

If you are travelling by taxi or private hire vehicle, your assistance dog should be allowed to travel with you under the Equality Act 2010. However, this does not apply if the driver has an exemption certificate, such as if they have an allergy to dogs; in such cases, the driver will have a 'notice of exemption' on their vehicle windscreen. Drivers are taught how to recognise assistance dogs and to welcome them into vehicles. It can help them to do this if your dog wears its harness or identification jacket whilst travelling, or if you carry your dog's identification card.

When travelling via coach or bus, it's worth finding out from the tour operator what accommodations will be available for you and your dog. Coaches come in many different layouts and seating and floor space can vary greatly. If you can, it helps to get your coach operator to reserve floor space for your dog in the seat next to you or to provide suitable space for your dog. It is also a good idea to tether your dog to a seat belt or seat stanchion using a car harness, to prevent them from sliding around in the event of an emergency stop. To help your dog feel more comfortable, you may wish to take a travel bed or blanket, a bowl, and a small supply of water in a travel bottle. If you are on a coach that is leaving mainland UK, you will need to find out what accommodations are available for your dog on the ferry or train on your crossing, especially where you can spend the dog prior to travel. Your dog ought to have regular rest breaks every 2-3 hours, so you may want to plan ahead depending on where your coach will stop on the journey. As for other modes of international travel, your dog will need to comply with the European Pets Travel Scheme (PETS); the PETS website has further information on the requirements you need to comply with.

If you are travelling via boat or ferry, you should be aware that not all ships or landing places are deemed suitable to accommodate assistance dogs; this may be due to safety considerations, staffing levels, or the suitability of passenger accommodation on the ship. If your dog cannot access a vessel, the travel operator should be able to provide further information as to why it is unsuitable to accommodate your dog. Operators are entitled to ask for evidence that an assistance dog has been trained by a recognised organisation, such as an ADUK charity or member of Assistance Dogs International (ADI). If the vessel is suitable for your dog, it can often help to notify the tour operator that you intend to travel with an assistance dog, ideally at least 48 hours prior to your departure.

318

Some cabins on cruise ships are very small, so there may be limited space for your dog. Larger cabins can be preferable but can cost considerably more and often need to be booked far in advance of your travel to secure them. On ferries, cabins can be booked for overnight crossings, but the number of cabins dedicated to passengers with assistance dogs may be limited, so it is worth booking your cabin space as early as you can. On some ferry journeys, dogs are sometimes expected to remain in the vehicle they are travelling on in the car deck. For most boats, though, you should be able to take your assistance dog onto the passenger deck of the vessel, although there may be some restrictions on where they can go due to safety measures. You can travel with your assistance dog on some cruise ships, but it's advisable to confirm with your operator that they are permitted prior to booking. Some operators will have dedicated spending areas for your dog on the passenger section of vessels, whilst others might expect you to keep your dog on the vehicle deck. In most cases, shipping operators expect you to manage any health-related issues that arise with your dog, such as sea sickness. It is therefore a good idea to have provisions in place to support your dog before taking it on a sea-faring vessel, and to be aware of the limitations of some cruise ships, destinations, or ports.

Travelling with an assistance dog may seem daunting at first, especially if is this is your first time navigating travel and working in unfamiliar places and conditions as a partnership. Planning the steps of your journey ahead of time or even creating an itinerary of appropriate rest stops can help you to feel a bit more confident and in control. Keeping in contact with your tour operator or booking agent is a great idea, as is giving them as much information and advance notice as possible that you'll be travelling with an assistance dog and finding out what support is available.

Travelling with a disability

There are so many options available to travel with all kinds of disabilities. When you first acquire a disability, chronic illness, or neurodivergent condition, travelling – and especially travelling alone or independently – might seem like an insurmountable feat. My advice would be to plan your journey out in advance, figure out what support you need, and liaise with your travel operator to keep them in the loop and to ensure that they can offer you the right support for your needs. This can help you to feel more prepared and confident to tackle your journey, as you know what to expect at each step of the way. Travelling with a disability can unfortunately take more planning and forethought, but the more you do it successfully, the more your confidence will grow.

Public and private modes of transport are only one factor when travelling around the UK, though. There are several other tips and tricks which I've learned over the years which can help when you're planning an outing or visiting an attraction. Let's have a quick look, and hopefully one of these tips will come in handy for you too.

Visiting attractions in the UK

We all enjoy visiting attractions for days out or when on holiday, and many attractions offer different options for disabled people, such as companion or carer tickets either for free or at a reduced cost. It's worth checking out the website for the attraction you're interested in visiting, to see if they offer these kinds of discounts and if there is any evidence you need to provide, such as a PIP letter or a Blue Badge. Certain venues – such as theme parks – may also offer priority access to attractions for disabled people to cut down on waiting times and to offer reasonable adjustments. Once again, it can help to check out the attraction's website to see what is on offer for disabled people and to see if you can book support or discounted tickets in advance of your trip.

Some types of venue offer their own schemes for disabled people. The UK Cinema Association (UKCA) and its member cinemas are striving to make visiting the cinema more inclusive and enjoyable for all. They are working to identify the barriers that disabled people face when going to the cinema, with the hope of removing these obstacles. They therefore offer the **Cinema CEA card.** Some disabled people need to be accompanied by carers or companions to enjoy the cinema experience, and the CEA card scheme allows the card holder to be accompanied by someone free of charge when they purchase a ticket at a participating cinema. The hope is that this will make visiting the cinema more accessible and inclusive for all.

321

As a disabled person, you may be eligible for **Purpl discounts** too. Purpl helps you to save money and was founded to offset the cost of living with a disability and help your money to go further. It was founded by someone who understands firsthand the challenges and costs of being disabled, and who puts the needs of the disabled people they support first. With Purpl, you can access great discounts from your favourite brands and get tailored deals sourced exclusively for the disabled community. They currently have over 90 brand partners and more coming. Purpl believes in giving back to disabled charities and so when you use their discount codes, you are supporting the disabled community too.

When visiting attractions across the UK, it's advisable to do your research and see what discounts and support you can access. But this does mean putting in the extra effort to find out whether places are accessible for your needs. Fortunately, though, there are a couple of apps that can help you here.

Apps to help with access

When you want to go anywhere as a disabled person, it can often feel like a lot of planning needs to go into even the smallest outing to make sure a venue is suitable for you and your access needs. Even then, the number of times I've been told that somewhere is wheelchair accessible only to turn up and find out that I need to traverse a flight of stairs or that there is in fact no ramp is frustrating. Thankfully, there are some handy apps out there which are designed to help disabled people to find accessible places more easily. **Sociability App** is one example of this. They believe that, for more than 1 billion disabled people worldwide, poor accessibility is a barrier to social inclusion and quality of life, and that knowing the accessibility of a venue beforehand can be transformative. Their mission is to organise the world's accessibility information and to give peace of mind to disabled people. The app allows you to explore venues and the adaptive features that they offer to find the places that are accessible to you. You can empower others by adding tags and photos whilst you are out to give even more accessibility information.

Another example of such an app is **AccessAble**, which seeks to take the chance out of going out. Originally called DisabledGo, the app was set up around 2000 by Dr Gregory Burke due to his own experiences as a wheelchair user and disabled walker; he was frustrated that when he searched for accessibility information about different locations, all he got was often a few unhelpful words. Today, trained surveyors check out every single place on the app in person to give accurate information. Their detailed access guide gives you in-depth information about the assistive features at a venue to help you to know in advance what it will be like when you visit and to work out if it will be accessible to you. All guides have Accessibility Symbols that give you a quick overview of what is available at the venue. All the collected information has been requested by the disabled community and their carers, and thousands of people are involved in collecting new information each year.

Both apps offer different things, and you ought to check out both to find the one that works best for you and your needs. Having these apps can help you to check access information in advance and plan ahead, so it's a good idea to consult them when you are preparing to visit somewhere. In addition to the support already offered, there are other ways to signal to staff at venues that you need a little extra support, such as via the Sunflower lanyard scheme.

The Hidden Disabilities Sunflower Lanyard Scheme[49]

Some disabilities, conditions, and chronic illnesses are not immediately obvious to others and are sometimes referred to as 'hidden', 'non-visible', 'invisible' or 'non-apparent' disabilities. For some people, this can make it hard for others to understand their condition and believe that someone with a non-apparent disability really does need support.

The Hidden Disabilities sunflower was created to encourage inclusivity, acceptance, and understanding for those with non-apparent conditions. The sunflower symbol is a tool for you to voluntarily share that you have a non-apparent disability. By

---

[49] Please note that all information was correct at time of publication [31 October 2025]. Please always check the Hidden Disabilities website for the most up-to-date information in cases of changes to this scheme.

wearing the sunflower symbol, you're letting others know that you might need extra support, understanding, or just some additional time. The sunflower was chosen for its distinctive appearance, because it is visible from a distance and because it is joyful and dynamic; it suggests happiness, positivity, growth, strength, and confidence, and is now a widely recognised symbol across the globe for non-apparent disabilities. Since its launch in 2016, businesses from every sector have been joining the global sunflower network. The sunflower symbol has now been launched in many countries worldwide, including Australia, Latin America, and the USA.

You can find out more information about the sunflower scheme, as well as purchase sunflower lanyards and symbols, on their website. If you have any accessibility needs, or if you have a disability that might not be easily apparent to others, it might be worth looking into the Sunflower scheme to make your needs more visible to others and to ensure that you get the support you need.

Some final thoughts...

We've covered a lot in this chapter, from getting mobility aids and assistance dogs, to navigating different transport systems, and looking at top tips for visiting attractions as a disabled person in the UK. Getting a mobility aid can sometimes be perceived as something negative – such as that you are 'giving up' on your remaining mobility – but this is often far from the truth. Mobility aids actually enable us to maintain our independence and give us more mobility, freedom, and options to engage with the world than we would have without them. For many, getting a sorely needed mobility aid is a liberating journey. There is no singular 'right time' to get a mobility aid, you just need to roll with it and go with what feels right for you.

A key benefit of mobility aids is that they help us to navigate the world around us. There is also a lot of support in place to help disabled people to access different places and modes of transport. Having a disability might add some extra planning and time into your journey, but it's always beneficial to look up access information or learn about any discounts that your destination offers for disabled people and their caring companions. When I first acquired my wheelchair, I worried about using it and about other people's perceptions, such as whether they'd think I was simply 'giving up' and resorting to the wheelchair instead of fighting for my remaining mobility. It felt uncomfortable to use adjustments too, such as the free carer ticket for many attractions. I nevertheless came to understand that only *my* opinions of my chair mattered and that these adjustments available on travel networks and at venues were there to give me equitable access compared to non-disabled people. My advice would be to stop worrying about whether you're 'disabled enough' and take advantage of the things that are there to help you!

What I learned:

- Despite what non-disabled people might think, mobility aids are freedom, joy, and independence!

- Getting a mobility aid is a personal decision, and there is no right or wrong time to get one. However, if you've been thinking that a mobility aid *might* help you, odds are it probably will, so go out and get it!

- There are so many kinds of mobility aids out there. Don't hesitate to shop around, try them all out, and weigh up the pros and cons of each before you make your decision. Mobility aids can be quite the financial investment!

- Personalising your mobility aid to match your personality can make you feel more confident when you're using it, so don't be afraid to go all out with stickers, washi tapes, spray paint, and sparkles!

- Welcoming an assistance dog into your life can be truly transformative, but it is a big responsibility too. Take time to do your research and consider whether you would prefer to owner-train or wait for an ADUK-trained dog, so that you can choose the path which is right for you.

- Know your rights on public transport, as you never know when you might have to recite them to a reticent bus driver!

- If you can, request assistance in advance whenever you are travelling. It helps to take the stress out of travel if you know that support will already be in place when you arrive.

- Make the most of any discounts or offers that are available for disabled people on public transport or at attractions and venues across the UK. Free or discounted carer tickets can make travelling and days out far more affordable!

Reflection Time:

1. Are you experiencing any signs that a mobility aid might help your daily life? If so, which signs are you experiencing?

2. Depending on your needs, have you thought about which mobility aid(s) might suit you best, especially if you need different ones for different tasks? Have you done any further research on these devices or even tried any of them?

3. If you need a mobility aid, have you thought about how you want to acquire the aid you need? The NHS, charities, and Access to Work can help, depending on your circumstances.

4. How do you usually travel? Are there any steps you can take to make this more accessible for you, such as applying to the Motability Scheme or downloading the Passenger Assistance app for train travel? It might help to make a personalised travel plan.

5. Would a Hidden Disabilities sunflower lanyard help you when visiting public places, even just to signal to staff that you

might need extra support? They can be purchased via the Hidden Disabilities website: https://hdsunflower.com/uk/

Chapter 10
Living Life on Your Own Terms
Claiming your in(ter)dependence

So far, the preceding chapters have sought to help you understand your life and your identity as a disabled person, how disability impacts on your relationships, navigating work or education, or learning how to look after your mental health and wellbeing. In many ways, we have been working up towards the ultimate goal for many disabled and non-disabled people: gaining your independence. We often strive to become fully-fledged, independent adults, but we rarely stop to question what it actually *means* to be independent. Society tends to impart this stereotypical way of thinking about independence, which entails moving out of your parental or carer's home, getting a job, potentially going to university, living independently and paying the bills, and maybe even finding a partner to enjoy life with, before getting married, and eventually having children.

Whilst societal norms teach us that we should strive for this vision of independence, there are in fact many ways that we can become independent and, indeed, in*ter*dependent. This can look different or might happen on a different timescale for anyone, but this can be even more the case for disabled people. However you claim your independence is valid and just as monumental an achievement. It's just that sometimes, we must do things a little differently as disabled people. This final chapter will look at what gaining your independence might entail and contain some top tips for achieving this along the way. So, without further ado, let's dive in and help you to find the independence your heart desires.

SMART Goals

For many, the goal for independence is to live in your own home, either alone or with a partner or roommates, and to have financial independence from your parents or guardians. This goal is achievable for many disabled people, although you may need to make some changes to your living spaces or routines to succeed. But this is far from the only way to become independent, either as a disabled or a non-disabled person. For some, living in a supported living facility, but managing their own carer schedule, could be a form of independence. Others may have financial independence to choose how to spend or save their own income, whilst others may live, work with, and care for an assistance dog who helps them to maintain their independence.

Whatever your overall goal for independence, it can help to break it down into smaller SMART goals to help them to feel more manageable and achievable. You might be asking, though, what exactly are SMART goals? This stands for **specific, measurable, achievable, relevant,** and **time-bound** goals. You can use this method to help you to clarify your ideas, focus your efforts, and to use your time and resources effectively; all of this will increase your chances of achieving your goals and living the life you want. By using the SMART goal framework, you can define the steps you'll need to take and decide on the milestones that indicate you're making progress along the way. The specificity of SMART goals allows you to visualise them more easily, which can help you to stay on track and achieve your goals efficiently and effectively.

If you're new to SMART goals, it can take a bit of practice to get into setting them, so let's look at a few tips for this. The first task is to consider the type of goal you're hoping to achieve and **make it specific**. It might help to use clear definitions, concrete words, and to answer prompt questions such as who you want to achieve the goal with, what you want to achieve, what you need to succeed, and how you will go about achieving your goal. You will then want to make your goal **measurable** by expressing it in terms of quantity, size, amount, or duration. It might help to consider which elements of your goal you can use to measure your progress, and to ask yourself how you will know once you have succeeded. For example, if you are trying to transition from a supported living facility or your familial home to your own place, you might set an initial goal of spending a few nights or even a week there before building up the amount of time you spend there. Having something tangible to work towards will help you to track your progress, and to celebrate small wins along the way to boost your motivation.

When writing SMART goals, you must ensure that your goal is **achievable.** This step focuses on why your goal is important to *you* and what you can do to make sure that it is attainable. If your goal is to independently manage your carer rota, for instance, you may need to gain certain skills to achieve this goal; you may need to learn diary management, how to manage employees, or some financial skills to manage payments. The next step to SMART goals is to make them **relevant** by aligning them with your values and your long-term objectives. This will help you to avoid spending time on tasks that are not pertinent to your goal. Reminding yourself of how this goal will benefit you in the long run can emphasise its relevance to your position today and, in turn, inspire and motivate you to achieve it. Another important factor in a SMART goal is to make it **time bound**. Setting yourself a realistic end date of when you want to have achieved your goal can help to provide motivation. If you do not manage to complete your goal within the set timeframe, try not to be too hard on yourself. Instead, take this as an opportunity to review how realistic your goal was and whether there is anything further you need or additional skills you need to obtain to achieve it.

As well as the SMART steps, it can be beneficial to set **regular check-ins** whilst working towards your original goal. Creating your goal can be inspirational and give you a burst of energy and motivation, but this enthusiasm may fade over time. If you set progress checks, it can help you to stay on track with your goal and to celebrate the progress you have made. By **celebrating the**

incremental little wins, you can keep boosting your motivation, as achieving big goals inevitably takes time. SMART goals can therefore be a great tool to help you on your journey to independence and to enable you to achieve your long-term objectives, whatever they may be!

My journey to independence

When I first became significantly unwell at the start of my university degree, I had to take the difficult decision to interrupt my studies for a year to pursue diagnosis and treatment. During that year, though, I could barely leave my bed due to the chronic pain and other symptoms that I was experiencing, as I did not have access to the right aids and medical support to help me. At that time, I was struggling and reliant on the care of my parents as I found it nigh-on impossible to do many things for myself, including cook, bathe, or get around.

But I was eighteen years old, I had just had a taste of independence in the few short weeks I had spent at university, and I had a boyfriend with whom I was beginning to envisage a life together. I desperately wanted to live independently from my parents, in my own university flat where I could have my friends and boyfriend round, and where I could start building a life for myself. Lying in my bed, I would often dream and fantasize about it. But I didn't share this dream with anyone for a while. Given the direction that my life had recently taken, I feared facing the reality that I might never be well enough to live independently again.

One day, though, my hopes slipped out in a conversation with my mum. I expected her to give me a dose of realism and to tell me that my dreams weren't achievable at that point in time. To my surprise, though, she calmly picked up a pad of paper and a pen, sipped her cup of chamomile tea, and said, 'Ok, so what do you need to do to live independently at university?' Stuttering a little in shock, I began to list all the things that I could think of, and we kept going until I could think of no more. We then set about turning each one into a goal that I could work on during the year I had interrupted from my studies and ranked them from the easiest to achieve to the hardest. Throughout the next 10 months, I worked as hard as I could on my goals and celebrated the small wins with my mum, dad, and boyfriend when we achieved each one and could triumphantly cross it off the list. With each goal I achieved, it felt like my world was opening up that little bit more. When it was time to return to university, I was able to mostly live and study independently with the right support systems in place, and my life was unrecognisable from the one I had been leading only 10 months before.

As I've aged and developed further conditions, my disabilities have had a greater impact on my life. I have again had to contend with a change to my independence, for instance, I can no longer cook or clean my own home. But I have also learned to reframe what independence means to me. When I was younger, I believed that

335

independence meant doing everything for yourself and not relying on anyone for anything, just like the little red hen in the children's fable. I couldn't have been more wrong, though! I now feel that to live independently means to live the life that you design and choose for yourself. For me, that means living with my partner and my fur babies, where we all *interdependently* care for one another. As such, I no longer feel that 'independence' means not relying on anyone else. I rely on my partner and my family for physical care sometimes, just as my partner relies on me in turn for emotional, mental health, and administrative support. Whilst I need support in some areas, I am more independent in others, such as working a full-time job and maintaining financial independence. There are many ways to think about independence, and it does not mean doing everything alone; it instead entails a form of interdependence to work with others who can support you in making choices for your own life. Being disabled has taught me that independence often comes with this mutual reliance on others for support. At the end of the day, we are all interdependent when it comes to caring for one another – no-one truly does *everything* by themselves, as we all need one another. But if that enables us to live the life we want and choose, then that's just being human! After all, no one is *completely* independent, as we all have times when we need emotional or physical support from others.

Claiming your independence: Carers and PAs

Whilst in my teenage years I strove after the stereotypical view of 'independence' from the familial home, I now appreciate that there are so many more ways to live interdependently as a disabled person. This is especially the case if we remember that living independently doesn't mean that you must do or even manage everything by yourself. 'Independent living' is itself the idea that people should have the same choices and control over their lives as everyone else, including disabled people.

For many disabled people, 'independent living' means being supported by carers or personal assistants (PAs), who provide a range of services. A carer or PA might assist with personal care needs, help with practical domestic tasks or light housekeeping, support disabled individuals with sport or leisure activities, or offer friendship or companionship. Carers can support people out in the community, such as in care or supported living facilities, or in a disabled person's own home.

To start the process of getting a carer, you can ask for a carers assessment from your local council to work out exactly what kind of support you might need.[50] The council may help pay towards your care, but even if they do not, they will still carry out the assessment for you to determine the support you need. Following the

---

[50] Please note that all information was correct at time of publication [31 October 2025]. Please always check Government or local council websites for the most up-to-date information in cases of changes to this scheme.

assessment, you then have several options about how to hire carers. You can use an agency, who will typically supply a carer or PA to your home for a management fee. This means that the agency will be your carer's employer and will deal with things like their pay and contract for you, as well as employment rights like sick pay, annual leave, or misconduct. Agencies usually have a pool of carers, so they can send an alternative person if your usual carer is sick or on holiday. Using an agency can be a good option if you're unsure or would not feel confident about being an employer. On the other hand, it does give you less control over who you have as your PA as different members of staff may come to support you at different times. It may cost more too, as agencies will take a fee or percentage of your PA's wage to pay for the service they provide to you.

Alternatively, you could employ your own carer or PA directly without the help of an agency. In this case, you would be your carer's employer, which has both benefits and drawbacks. Employing a carer directly gives you choice over who will support you, rather than having to accept the person an agency might send. This means you can choose to have the same person or people caring for you consistently, and you can decide the hours you want them to work or the tasks you'd like them to complete. If you employ your own carer, though, you are responsible for their pay, contract, taxes, and employment rights like sick pay and holidays. You could, then, be without care if your only PA is sick or on holiday, whereas an agency would send someone to cover these shifts. The task of managing your team of PAs and dealing with any issues such as personality clashes or unprofessional conduct would also fall to you, which some people may find stressful.

To overcome these hurdles, some people use a mix of local authority support, agencies, and being their PAs employer to work out the best care package for them. This means that they can have some control over who they hire as a PA, but that the agency can send someone to provide care if your regular PA is unavailable. When you have your care assessment with the council, you might want to talk to your assessor about what options are available in your local area and think about what might suit you and your needs best. Some local authorities run services to help disabled people and potential PAs meet, so it might be worth asking them about any PA registers in your area. They may alternatively have a service that can put you in touch with other people who have employed a carer or personal assistant, so that you can learn more about it and ask them for advice.

There is no right or wrong answer when it comes to deciding how to manage your care; the most important thing is to find the solution that works best for *you*. You could create a list of must-haves, as well as a list of things you're willing to compromise on. You might want to consider factors such as budget, level of control, your confidence to manage admin, and what's available in your local area.

Whether you use an agency or become an employer, receiving care can be an incredibly intimate act. You are letting people you do not know well into your personal space and, in some cases, asking them to help you with some of the most personal tasks you can imagine. It can help to build up a relationship with your carers first, so that you both feel more comfortable around one another. Whilst building this relationship might seem somewhat artificial, there are nevertheless some things you can work on to start getting to know your carers:

- **Ask about their background**. Be inquisitive about your carer. Ask them their name and a bit about their background, such as how long they have been a personal assistant and what motivated them to come into this line of work. Your carer will likely appreciate you taking an interest in them as a person, beyond the requirements of their job.

- **Ask questions**. Whether you employ your carer directly or through an agency, you are still letting another person into your personal space. This will come with questions and concerns for both of you. Don't be afraid to talk to your carer to better understand their queries and concerns, as it's only by doing this that you can help to put them at ease.

- **Be open and honest**. Be open and honest about your needs and about your expectations of receiving care. This helps you to appreciate each other's perspectives and to find boundaries that you can mutually agree upon, so that you are both comfortable with the care you either give or receive.

- **Practice active listening.** Pay close attention to what your carer is saying and try to understand their perspective. Listen especially closely if they raise any concerns with you about their work and ask questions so that you can better understand the things which are causing them anxiety. Try to understand that this is not a criticism and instead keep an open mind and collaborate with your carer to work out a solution.

- **Communicate respectfully.** Be clear and direct in your communication with your carer, whilst remaining polite, considerate, and respectful. Remember that, whilst this relationship may give rise to a friendship over time, it is still a working relationship, and we all deserve to be treated respectfully and with consideration in our working lives.

- **Set clear boundaries.** In your first few meetings, it might help to establish what is expected of both you and your carer in this relationship to avoid misunderstandings and miscommunication. If you wish to formalise this, you could write up a contract or agreement to clearly set out the boundaries for you both.

- **Give positive feedback.** We all like to hear when we've done a good job on something, and it can help your relationship with your carer if you regularly express your appreciation for their efforts and hard work. If you do need to give them constructive feedback to help them improve on a task, it can help to start with some praise or a positive to soften the blow!

- **Respect one another's privacy.** Your carer may be helping you with intimate acts of personal care, or you may have a live-in carer who shares your home with you at times. To support a healthy working relationship, it's crucial that you respect one another's personal space and privacy.

- **Support your care worker to succeed.** Especially if you employ your carer directly, investing in their work and career can show that you are willing to support them. You can ask your care co-ordinator at the local authority for guidance on where you can get practical support or training for you and your carer. *Skills for Care* and *Carers UK* also have several useful guides if you are looking for help with this.

Receiving care enables many disabled people to live independently and thrive, and to have choice and control over their own lives. Having a care support package does not come without its own unique set of challenges, but there is plenty of support out there to help you to successfully manage your care. Perhaps the most important thing when it comes to receiving care is to find someone you feel comfortable with and with whom you can build a close working relationship, especially as receiving care can be an incredibly intimate act.

Supported Living Arrangements

Whilst most care packages are provided to disabled people in their own homes, there are yet more ways for you to live independently out in the community. One way is through supported or assisted living arrangements; this is a person-centred approach to housing and support which enables disabled people to live independently within their communities. Also known as sheltered housing, it provides another option for disabled people to live on their own terms whilst still receiving the support or care they need to thrive.

Unlike residential care, assisted living encourages autonomy, choice, and inclusion by providing flexible support that is tailored to each person's needs. Whilst residential care offers 24/7 support in a structured environment, supported living promotes individualised support and community integration to enable people to live full lives on their own terms. It therefore focuses on building independence, strengthening social connections, and achieving personal growth for disabled people. Support workers collaborate closely with each person to develop a personalised support plan, which is regularly reviewed to ensure that the disabled person is receiving the right support from key people in their life.

Assisted living arrangements are usually provided by local councils, charities, and commercial companies. The disabled person typically holds the tenancy agreement for their accommodation, thereby giving them legal rights and responsibilities as tenants.

Residents then receive the support and care that they need to live independently and to thrive. This might include support with tasks like dressing, washing, going to the toilet, or taking medication. On-site staff may provide meals, personal care, or domestic support. Eligibility for assisted living is determined by an assessment which considers the disabled person's needs and their financial situation. Residents with savings or investments over a certain threshold may be asked to privately fund their place.

Taking up a place in an assisted living facility can have many benefits. The personalised care available in these facilities provides tailored support to each person, allowing them to maintain as much independence as possible. Assisted living facilities further offer social interaction, as residents can participate in planned activities and socialise with one another, which combats isolation and promotes mental wellbeing. For those with support needs, assisted living offers a sense of safety and security for the disabled person and their loved ones, especially knowing that features like emergency call systems, monitored access, and round-the-clock staff are available. There may even be on-site healthcare facilities and medical professionals readily available. Even if you do not live in an assisted living facility, you can still receive support from them. Some facilities offer short-term respite places for family care-givers, which can in turn reduce stress and the possibility of burn out.

Whilst assisted living facilities can bring many benefits, there are a few other things that you might wish to consider in more depth. As a disabled person, transitioning into an assisted living facility may result in feeling a loss of control over daily routines and decision making to a certain degree, as these facilities have some routines and restrictions to ensure they can care for everyone, such as set mealtimes. Depending on the facility, assisted living can be incredibly expensive too. Certain options might be financially out of reach, or you may have to fundraise or apply for grants to enable you to live in one of these facilities. It's worth noting that not all facilities provide the same level of care, so it can help to do your own careful research before deciding to enter a facility or securing a place for a loved one, so that you can be sure that quality standards are met. Whilst facilities often arrange social activities for the residents, there is still a risk of social isolation if an individual does not or cannot participate. Assisted living facilities may further have limited privacy for individuals, especially if there are shared living spaces. Finally, adapting to an assisted living facility can be incredibly stressful and may require a period of acclimatisation for disabled people and their families.

Whilst assisted living facilities can be a great option for those with care and support needs to live independently, it can be a big adjustment for disabled people and their families. Although assisted living promotes autonomy and social integration, these things still need careful co-ordination and induction if they are to be successful.

Before deciding on an assisted living facility, it can be worth exploring all options in terms of receiving care and support within the home. For some, though, assisted living facilities enable them to thrive and live independently within the community, leading the life they choose.

Tips for living independently with a disability[51]

When I first tried to live independently as a disabled person and wheelchair user, it felt like I was having to figure everything out for the first time again. Not just in terms of day-to-day tasks like getting dressed or bathing, I also felt totally lost amidst the systems that were there to support me. It was incredibly overwhelming, and I struggled for many years before receiving the support that I could have accessed from the start. The reality, though, is that there is support out there if you are a disabled person trying to live independently – you just need to reach out and make the most of it. The following sections will look at different kinds of support that might be available to either help you financially or to help you to live independently as a disabled person.

---

[51] Please note that all information in this section was correct at time of publication [31 October 2025]. Please always check Government, NHS, and other websites for the most up-to-date information in cases of changes to this scheme.

Free NHS Prescriptions and Delivery

NHS prescriptions can be expensive, particularly if you are on regular medication, as the prices just keep going up year on year. Some people are automatically entitled to free NHS prescriptions under the medical exemption certificate. Full details can be found on the NHS website, but you can apply for medical exemption if, for example, you have diabetes, hypoparathyroidism, epilepsy, cancer, various other conditions, or a continuing physical disability which means you cannot go out without the help of another person. You can apply for exemption through a form available via your GP practice.

If you do not qualify for free prescriptions under the disability criteria, it might be worth applying for a prescription prepayment certificate. You can purchase them for either 3 or 12 months online and spread the cost by paying monthly. If you take several regular medications, the savings from a prepayment certificate can be considerable.

Several pharmacies nowadays offer a delivery service for your repeat prescriptions. Pharmacy2U, Well, and Lloyds all offer schemes where your regular repeat prescriptions can be delivered to your door at a time that suits you. This can be a great option for those with regular prescriptions who have limited mobility or who might struggle to get out and about. Pharmacy apps have features where you can set reminders to refill your prescriptions too, and so it can help with medical admin and make your prescriptions one less thing to worry about.

Council Tax Reduction

Depending on your disability and your needs, you may be eligible to apply for a council tax discount or reduction if you or someone you live with is disabled. For instance, you might qualify for the scheme if you live in a larger property than you would need if you or the other person were not disabled, such as needing extra room for a wheelchair. You will need to show that you have an extra bathroom, kitchen, or other room that you need for the disabled person, or extra space inside your property, such as wider doors or walkways for using a wheelchair. The property must be the main home for at least one disabled person, whether an adult or child, although they do not have to be responsible for paying the council tax bill. If you are eligible for the scheme, your bill will be reduced to the next lowest council tax band.

Occupational Therapists and Home Improvements

If you own or rent a property as a disabled person and need some adjustments to live there safely, you might be able to access help through your local council's occupational therapy service. Occupational therapists (OTs) help you to improve your ability to undertake daily tasks and participate in meaningful activities. Your council may have a service where one of their OTs will come to your home and undertake a free assessment to determine the kind of support you need and suggest any aids or home adaptations which could be made to help you.

The support that OTs offer might include things like widening or lowering steps, installing grab rails, creating ramps and lifts, adding a stairlift, lowering kitchen countertops, or widening doorways. OTs may recommend aids such as commodes, perch stools, adapted cutlery, long-handled loofahs, or shoehorns, to name but a few. Your council should pay for each adaptation to your home which costs less than £1,000. For more expensive modifications, such as building a wet room or widening doors, you may need to self-fund or look at other funding options to cover these costs.

In the first instance, you might be able to apply to your council for a **Disabled Facilities Grant**.[52] This will not affect any benefits you get, and how much you receive will usually depend on your household income and any savings over £6,000. In England, you can receive a Disabled Facilities Grant of up to £30,000, although some councils may award more. Depending on your income, though, you may need to pay something towards the cost of the work at your property. Another option is to apply to **Independence at Home** for

---

[52] Please note that all information in this section was correct at time of publication [31 October 2025]. Please always check Government and local council websites for the most up-to-date information in cases of changes to this scheme.

help towards the costs of making home adaptations due to your disability.[53] Independence at Home is a charity which provides grants to people of all ages who have a physical or learning disability, or a long-term illness, and who are in financial need. The financial aid they provide enables grant recipients to purchase mobility and disability equipment or home adaptations to have an immediate, practical, and positive impact on their lives and increase their independence. There may be other charities and organisations out there who offer grants for costly home adaptations, so it's worth doing your research and making applications where you can.

Capped Water Bills

If you are disabled, you can apply for the **WaterSure** scheme to help with your water bills. To apply, you must be on benefits, have a water meter, and need to use lots of water for medical reasons. Some water companies also offer the scheme if you're on Disability Living Allowance or Personal Independence Payment, so it's worth checking with your supplier. If you receive help from the WaterSure scheme, your water bill will be capped; this means that you will not pay any more than the average metered bill for the area that your water company services. If your normal water bill is less than the

---

[53] Please note that all information in this section was correct at time of publication [31 October 2025]. Please always check the Independence at Home charity website for the most up-to-date information in cases of changes to this scheme.

company's WaterSure cap anyway, you will only be billed for the water that you use.

Priority Service Register

Electricity, gas, and water supply companies must ensure that their services are accessible to you as a disabled person. There are many ways that they can support you when you're on the **Priority Services Register (PSR)**. The PSR is free to join and helps utility companies to support customers who have additional communication, access, or safety needs. You are eligible if you have a disability or chronic illness, are d/Deaf or hard of hearing, are blind or partially sighted, or if you have a mental health or neurodivergent condition. If you are on the PSR, you will receive extra support from utility companies such as providing information in accessible formats, notice of planned cuts or supply issues, help with meter readings and bill payments, and priority support in an emergency. It's free to sign up to the register and you can do this online by searching 'priority services register' to access the PSR website.

TV Licensing

Disabled people may be eligible for a 50% reduction of their TV license. If you are blind or partially sighted, or if you live with someone who is, you can apply for the discount. The licence must be in the blind or partially sighted person's name, though. You can

351

apply for the discount online and will need to provide documents as proof of your disability.

Technologies to help with independent living

Disability has heavily influenced the world of technology, especially over the last few decades. From electric toothbrushes to computer keyboards or easy-grip kitchenware, the odds are that you will likely have a piece of technology in your home that has been designed with disabled people in mind. Technologies, apps, and assistive software nowadays enable disabled people to live, work, socialise, and enjoy their leisure time independently, and there are several different technologies out there to suit all kinds of accessibility needs.

Assistive technology describes devices and software which help disabled people to live more independently, whether in their work, education, or daily lives. It includes things like screen readers, adaptive keyboards, alternative input devices, Braille displays, or screen magnifiers, to name a few. Another kind of assistive technology includes **alternative input devices**. Not everyone can use a mouse and keyboard to operate a computer, so alternative input devices give disabled people different options to use a computer in a way that works best for them. This might be via head pointers, foot switches, sip and puff devices, eye-tracking software, or text-to-speech software. Other disabled people may use **augmentative and**

352

alternative communication, or AAC, to communicate with others in their personal and professional lives. AAC incorporates a range of tools to help people who are non-verbal or who otherwise struggle to communicate. Perhaps one of the most famous examples of AAC was the device used by renowned physicist Stephen Hawking.

There are also numerous technologies which support blind and partially sighted people to thrive and lead independent lives. There are **Braille notetakers** or refreshable tactile **Braille displays** which convert digital text on screen into Braille. **Dictation software** is now available on computers, smartphones, and tablets and can both convert speech into text and carry out commands. **Screen reader software** is now readily available on electronic devices and reads everything on the screen aloud for blind or partially sighted users; this software can further work with braille display devices to convert on-screen information into a readable format.

Beyond these devices, there are several other aids which can help blind and partially sighted people to thrive around the home. Many people find that it helps to put **Bumpons** – which are small adhesive dots or squares – on things like their microwaves or ovens to highlight key functions or commonly used cooking temperatures. **Talking scales, jugs, or liquid-level indicators** can all help when preparing a meal in the kitchen. The **PenFriend** audio labeller might come in handy too. It allows you to record audio information which you can then play back by getting the PenFriend to read a label. You could attach these labels to condiments in your fridge or outfits in your wardrobe; the PenFriend would then recount the details of your outfits or the contents of the condiments as you recorded them, allowing you to make choices independently. If you're looking for aids that might help you as a blind or partially sighted person, the Royal National Institute of Blind People (RNIB) has an online shop where you can search for all the aids available which might help you to live more independently.

Whatever your disability, the growth in **smart home technology** has had a tremendous impact on the lives of disabled people and, in many cases, helps them to live more independently. These technologies could make your daily life easier, from controlling your lighting and heating to seeing who is at the door and setting up home security. Smart home technology could help with lighting, temperature, security, cooking, telling time and setting reminders, TV and radio, laundry, or entertainment and gaming systems – the possibilities are endless! There are so many different smart home technologies out there, so it is a good idea to do your research to find out which one(s) will be best for the tasks you need them to do. You can control these systems using a smartphone, tablet, computer or even voice-activated hubs such as the Google Nest, Amazon Echo, or Apple HomePod. If you want to use a voice-activated hub, you will need to make sure that you buy accessories which are compatible with it, such as compatible smart plugs.

If you are interested in setting up a smart home system, or other technology in your home, but are not the most tech-savvy, there is help available. **AbilityNet** has volunteers who provide free IT support to disabled people in their own homes. They can help with choosing or setting up a smart home system or a computer or a tablet. They can assist with specialist computer aids or adaptations, as well as technical problems with software, hardware or the internet.

Useful Apps

In addition to technological devices, there are many applications available on Android devices and iPhones which can help to remove some of the barriers that disabled people continue to face in their lives. Many entertainment apps – such as **Netflix, Amazon Prime Video,** or **BBC iPlayer** – have subtitles available for their programmes. **Subtitle Viewer!** for Apple devices shows subtitles on your phone for TV shows or movies that do not otherwise have subtitles. Certain apps can help you transcribe your phone calls into text. **Roger Voice** adds captions to voice and video conversations in real time. Other apps allow you to take live transcription of what is being said around you. It's important to ask permission from the people you want to record before you record them. To see if this kind of app could be useful, you could try **Google Live Transcribe, Otter,** or **Glean**.

There are also apps which have been designed with blind or partially sighted people in mind, especially ones which help you to better understand your surroundings. **Be My Eyes** is a popular app

355

in this vein. It connects you to a volunteer via live video call, who can then help you with tasks such as checking expiry dates, distinguishing colours, reading instructions, or describing and navigating new surroundings. **BlindSquare** is another app which describes the environment and announces points of interest as you travel, such as shops, restaurants, or street crossings. **Navilens** helps blind or partially sighted people to explore their surroundings. The app is free to use and gives the user information about the environment around them through strategically placed Navilens codes which can be read by a smartphone. Navilens codes can be placed in the environment around us - such as in subways, on buildings, or on buses - or they could be incorporated onto product packaging to convey important information.

Just as there are apps to help those with low vision, there are certain apps which have been designed with d/Deaf or hard of hearing people in mind. **ExSilent's HearYouNow** app was created by a manufacturer of hearing aids and supports those with hearing loss who are not yet ready to use hearing aids. The app amplifies sounds and is highly adjustable to adapt to a range of hearing needs to help users to better understand the sounds around them. The volume is adjustable per ear and users can replay sounds whilst controlling the volume.

There are so many apps which can help with the daily symptoms and admin involved in living with a disability or chronic illness. For instance, whilst sleep hygiene is without a doubt important, certain apps can help with relaxation and getting better quality sleep. **BetterSleep** is designed to improve sleep quality and overall wellbeing by providing a range of tools, content, and features aimed at developing healthy sleep habits. **Headspace** is a personal favourite of mine, as they aim to provide everyone with access to mental health support through evidence-based meditation and mindfulness tools. The app helps you to create life-long habits to support your mental health and find a happier and healthier you. **Calm** is another great option which seeks to improve your overall health and happiness. It can help you to improve your sleep quality, reduce stress and anxiety, and work on self-improvement.

There is a further range of apps aimed at supporting disabled people with chronic pain and managing medical and emergency information. **Curable** has a virtual pain coach called Clara, which uses a biopsychosocial approach to pain and interacts with you by sending messages, activities, and resources to help you to better manage your pain. It was created by people who live with chronic pain themselves, so it can feel like you're talking to someone who truly gets it. **In Case of Emergency (ICE)** is a must-have app for anyone who might need regular emergency care. It stores your personal and medical information in the app, which first responders and others can then access if you are unable to share it directly. You can also set up the app to send messages to your loved ones or emergency contacts when you're in an urgent situation. Finally, **Medisafe app** can be useful for disabled or chronically ill people who tend to have a lot of prescriptions. It is a medicine reminder app that is simple to use and which helps you to track your medications, reminding you when it's time to order a refill.

Technologies and apps can revolutionise your life with a disability by making daily tasks easier or helping you to regain your independence. There are so many different technologies and aids out there, with more being developed each day, and so things are continually improving for people with disabilities. If you want to live more independently, it's worth looking at what technologies and apps might help to support you and facilitate a life with greater independence. What's especially noteworthy is that many technologies which were originally conceptualised for disabled people have since been adopted by non-disabled people and brought into the mainstream, offering fantastic examples of accessibility benefitting everyone.

Some final thoughts…

As a disabled person, there is no right way that your life or claiming your independence needs to take. Your independence is defined by *you* and the things that you can do and want to achieve in your life. Being independent may mean being free to choose how to spend your time or being free to manage your own carer timetable and employees. Needing help from others for your care or support needs makes you no less independent. Quite the opposite! Receiving care might be what *enables* you to live the most independent life possible for you.

My advice would be to try not to measure 'independence' by the arbitrary and stereotypical standards that society often sets. Independence looks different for us all and, at different times throughout our lives, we're all dependent on the care of others for things. Independence could entail living completely on your own, or it might mean having carers to support you, or living in an assisted living facility. All are valid options when it comes to claiming your independence as a disabled person.

Whatever your goal for your independence, try to set yourself SMART goals to have measurable and achievable targets that you can work towards. Keep track of your progress and keep celebrating the little wins to keep up that motivation which will spur you on. Remember as well that, when it comes to claiming your independence, you do not have to do this alone. There is so much support out there to help you live independently and thrive as a disabled person, so get out there and make the most of it!

What I learned:

- There are so many ways to think about what it means to be independent, especially as a disabled person. Think carefully about what living independently looks like for you.

- Setting SMART goals towards living independently can be a great way to build up slowly and increase your confidence with the small wins.

- Being independent doesn't mean that you must do *everything* for yourself, or by yourself, all the time. Remember, we are all human and we all need to rely on the care of others at certain times in our lives.

- Being independent means living the life you choose for yourself.

- There are some benefits to being disabled, such as free NHS prescriptions, council tax reductions, or capped water bills. It's worth it to do your research and see what you may be entitled to.

- Technology can be a great help to live independently as a disabled person. There is a plethora of different assistive devices, smart home technology, and software out there, so it's a good idea to do your research to see what might make your life easier.

Reflection Time

1. Do you feel that the SMART goal model would help you set goals towards your independence? If so, are there any SMART goals that you would like to set? It can help to work through each step individually.

2. What does independence look like for you? Do you want to rent or buy your own home, or do you need carers/ personal

assistants to support you? Would supported living offer you greater independence?

3. If you need carers/ personal assistants, have you thought about whether you would like to be their employer, whether you would like to use an agency, or whether you use a mix of both?

4. Which technologies and apps might be most useful for you to live independently?

Rolling With It

Congratulations, you've made it to the end of the book! I hope that you've found something useful in it and that it has been helpful to you living as a disabled person. With any luck, you now feel more prepared to tackle all that life with a disability can throw at you.

I thought it would be useful here to sum up the main things that I have learned over the decades that I've lived with my disability, in the hope that it gives you a bit of a short-cut on your own journeys. So, here goes. I want you to know that it's perfectly natural to grieve the life you thought you'd have without disability in the picture; it doesn't make you ungrateful for what you still do have, it makes you *human*. But please don't grieve forever, as you will miss out on the rest of what this beautiful life has to offer. At some point, you just have to roll with it and make the most of the hand that life has dealt you.

Another thing I've learned is that it's normal to struggle with accepting your disability as part of your identity. When I first became disabled, I was angry and didn't want my disability to have anything to do with my life or how I saw myself. Again, though, try not to fight this identity struggle too much. Once you've become disabled, your disability will affect pretty much every aspect of your life and influence how you experience the world around you. By rolling with it and accepting disability as part of your identity, you will find an inner peace and acceptance. At the same time, though, remember that you are so much more than *just* your disability and that it is not your whole identity. Try to still find time and space in your life for the things you love and remain open to new passions that will continue to shape who you are as you grow.

Living with a disability has taught me a lot about myself, but I have also learned a lot about my relationships with other people too. Your relationships will inevitably change once you become disabled. Some will strengthen, whilst others will fade away. Losing friends can be immensely difficult but remember that it's ok to let go of relationships that are hurting you or that are no longer serving your needs. Disability is not just about losing friendships, though. Perhaps one of the greatest gifts of becoming disabled is that you will become part of the wonderful disability community, which can be a source of true understanding, validation, and lifelong friendship, if you open yourself to its possibilities.

As well as the friendships which sustain us, finding romantic partner(s) with whom you can share everything is one of life's sweetest pleasures. Although dating with a disability does bring its own plethora of challenges, never let anyone make you feel unworthy of love because you are disabled. You are an amazing, interesting, empathetic, and caring person, and someone that anyone would be lucky to date. Dating with a disability can be hard at times but know that there are so many fantastic people out there who are ready to love you for *you*, your disability included.

363

For anyone who becomes disabled, it won't take you long to realise that we sadly do not live in an accessible world, nor do we live in one without ableism, discrimination, or medical gaslighting. This is why, as disabled people, we can't be shy but must stand up for ourselves and let our voices be heard! You will need to learn to be your own self-advocate and speak up for your rights and needs. As hard and as isolating as this can feel sometimes, remember too that you are not alone in this fight. The disability community will stand behind you and can be a source of strength and solidarity, as can the ever-expanding network of disability allies ready to take up your cause if you need them.

As much as I have tried to remain positive in this book – and in my general outlook on life – I cannot lie to you. Being disabled is incredibly hard sometimes, and especially when you must continually advocate just to receive your basic human rights. This is why it is of such importance to look after your physical and mental health and wellbeing when you are disabled. Disability brings its own challenges in this domain too but always remember that you are deserving of self-care and nurturing your own wellbeing. And something I definitely wish I'd learned sooner is that there is no shame in asking for professional help when you need it, despite what the voice of your internalised ableism might try to tell you!

Thinking about our day-to-day lives, education and employment often feature heavily and can also give our lives meaning and purpose. Whichever path you choose, know that there is support out there to help you as a disabled person navigating work or education. You might need to be your own self-advocate, though, and be proactive in pursuing the support you need. As a disabled person, you can rarely just wait for people to come to you – you've got to go out and get what you need! Luckily, there are so many kinds of aids nowadays to support you. They rarely come cheap, though, which is just another way in which society makes it harder to live in this world as a disabled person. I wish I'd known sooner that it quite literally pays to do your research into which aid(s) are right for you and how you can get them funded. Whilst mobility aids can be transformative, there is sadly still a lot of internalised ableism that persists when it comes to deciding if you need an aid. Try to challenge these thoughts and unlearn this internalised ableism, as I guarantee you will feel a lot better afterwards! And when it comes to aids, if you think that one would help you, odds are that you're probably right, as *you* know *your* body best.

Now we're getting to the deep stuff. In our society, it often feels like there is a script of how life is *supposed* to play out. At eighteen, you head off to university and get a degree, and maybe you find a partner along the way. You then get married, build your career, buy a house, and eventually have kids. There are disabled people who lead this life, but I've learned that – as a disabled woman – it's ok to go off-script and live life on your own terms. Being disabled has taught me that it's ok to just roll with it in life, rather than planning every little thing. Life is what you make it and there are so many ways to live this life which bring us joy, and that is the main goal we should aim for in our life.

Being disabled in this messed-up but beautiful and amazing world comes with all kinds of challenges and curve balls that you must face. But, at the same time, facing these challenges has given rise to the greatest gift that my disability has given me: a new perspective on life that I term 'rolling with it'. The unpredictable nature of living with a disability has taught me that – just as my wheelchair keeps me rolling along – I just need to roll with it in life to keep things moving. When you roll with it, the difficulties and hard parts of being disabled bring you down less, as you know that you'll eventually roll on by to find joy again. Given this unpredictability of life, it is perhaps also better not to have preconceptions of what your life can or should be. Rather, life has many ways of surprising us and we might discover important things about ourselves when we roll with it and remain open to discovery. Rolling with life as a disabled person has taught me to enjoy what life has to offer, to find joy in the small moments, and to let yourself be surprised. Essentially, life happens *for* you when you just roll with it!

www.ingramcontent.com/pod-product-compliance
Lightning Source LLC
Chambersburg PA
CBHW071704120626
46550CB00001B/101